Immunology at a Glance

Immunology at a Glance

J. H. L. PLAYFAIR
Professor of Immunology
Middlesex Hospital Medical School
London

SECOND EDITION

BLACKWELL SCIENTIFIC PUBLICATIONS
OXFORD LONDON EDINBURGH BOSTON MELBOURNE

First published 1979
Reprinted 1980
Second edition 1982
Reprinted 1983

Set by Getset Ltd
Eynsham, Oxon,
printed and bound in Great Britain
by Billing & Sons Limited
Guildford, London, Oxford, Worcester

DISTRIBUTORS

USA
  Blackwell Mosby Book Distributors
  11830 Westline Industrial Drive
  St Louis, Missouri 63141

Canada
  Blackwell Mosby Book Distributors
  120 Melford Drive, Scarborough
  Ontario, M1B 2X4

Australia
  Blackwell Scientific Book
  Distributors
  214 Berkeley Street, Carlton
  Victoria 3053

British Library
Cataloguing in Publication Data
  Playfair, J H L
      Immunology at a glance
      1. Immunology
      I. Title
      616.07'9   QR181

  ISBN 0-632-00805-9

Preface

This is not a textbook for immunologists, who already have plenty of excellent ones to choose from. Rather, it is aimed at all those whose work immunology impinges on, but who may hitherto have lacked the time to keep abreast of a subject that can sometimes seem impossibly fast-moving and intricate.

Yet everyone with a degree in medicine or the biological sciences is already familiar with a good deal of the basic knowledge required to understand immunological processes, often needing no more than a few quick blackboard sketches to see roughly how they work. This is a book of sketches which have proved useful over the years, recollected (and artistically touched up) in tranquility.

The Chinese sage who remarked that one picture was worth a thousand words was certainly not an immunology teacher, or his estimate would not have been so low! In this book the text has been pruned to the minimum necessary for understanding the figures, omitting almost all historical and technical details, which can be found in the larger textbooks listed on the next page. In trying to steer a middle course between absolute clarity and absolute up-to-dateness, I am well aware of having missed both by a comfortable margin. But even in immunology, what is brand-new does not always turn out to be right, while the idea that any form of presentation, however unorthodox, will make simple what other authors have already shown to be complex can only be, in Dr Johnson's heartfelt words, 'the dream of a philosopher doomed to wake a lexicographer'. My object has merely been to convince workers in neighbouring fields that modern immunology is not quite as forbidding as they may have thought.

It is perhaps the price of specialisation that some important aspects of nature lie between disciplines and are consequently ignored for many years (transplant rejection is a good example). It follows that scientists are wise to keep an eye on each others' areas so that in due course the appropriate new disciplines can emerge — as immunology itself did from the shared interests of bacteriologists, haematologists, chemists, and the rest.

Acknowledgements

My largest debt is obviously to the immunologists who made the discoveries this book is based on; if I had credited them all by name it would not have been a slim volume. In addition, I am grateful to my colleagues at the Middlesex Hospital for information, advice, and criticism at all stages, particularly Dr J. Brostoff, Dr V. Eisen, Dr F.C. Hay, Dr P. Lydyard, Dr S. Marshall-Clarke, and Professor I.M. Roitt. My secretary, Miss Philippa Peck, and Mr R.R. Phillips and his colleagues in the photographic department of the Middlesex Hospital, worked tirelessly to get the manuscript and the figures right. I then showed the draft to Dr H.E.M. Kay, Professor C.A. Mims, and Professor L. Wolpert all of whom made valuable suggestions for improvement. My son Edward supplied a useful undergraduate view. Finally I would like to thank Per Saugman of Blackwell Scientific Publications for his encouragement in the first place.

Note on the second edition

Two years is a long time in immunology, and almost all sections of this book have had to be brought up to date. I have also taken the opportunity to correct some errors and omissions, in which I was helped, as always, by my colleagues at the Middlesex, to whom should be added Dr A. Cooke and Dr D. Male. Perhaps the biggest advances in recent years have been in the understanding of the immunoglobulin genes; this section has been entirely rewritten. However it will no doubt go out of date again equally quickly — which is the sort of thing that makes immunology perenially fascinating.

How to use this book

Each of the figures (listed opposite) represents a particular topic, corresponding roughly to a 45-minute lecture. Newcomers to the subject may like first to read through the **text** (left-hand pages), using the figures only as a guide; this can be done at a sitting.

Once the general outline has been grasped, it is probably better to concentrate on the **figures** one at a time. Some of them are quite complicated and can certainly not be taken in 'at a glance', but will need to be worked through with the help of the **legends** (right hand pages), consulting the **index** for further information on individual details; once this has been done carefully they should subsequently require little more than a cursory look to refresh the memory.

It will be evident that the figures are highly diagrammatic and not to scale; indeed the scale often changes several times within one figure. For an idea of the actual sizes of some of the cells and molecules mentioned, refer to **Appendix I**.

The reader will also notice that examples are drawn sometimes from the mouse, in which useful animal so much fundamental immunology has been worked out, and sometimes from the human, which is after all the one that matters. Luckily the two species are, from the immunologist's viewpoint, remarkably similar.

Further reading

I cannot do better than recommend the textbooks I myself consult regularly, and which largely furnished the raw material for this book.

Alexander J.W. & Good R.A. *Fundamentals of Clinical Immunology*. W.B. Saunders, Philadelphia, London, 1977 (338 pp).

Fudenberg H.H., Stites D.P., Caldwell J.L. & Wells J.V. (eds) *Basic and Clinical Immunology*, 2nd edn. Lange Medical Publications, Los Altos, California, 1978 (758 pp).

Gell P.G.H., Coombs R.R.A. & Lachmann P.J. (eds) *Clinical Aspects of Immunology*, 3rd edn. Blackwell Scientific Publications, Oxford, 1975 (1754 pp).

McConnell I., Munro A. & Waldman H. *The Immune System*, 2nd edn. Blackwell Scientific Publications, Oxford, 1981 (352 pp).

Mims C.A. *The Pathogenesis of Infectious Disease*. Academic Press, London, 1976 (246 pp).

Park B.H. & Good R.A. *Principles of Modern Immunobiology*. Lea and Febiger, Philadelpia, 1974 (617 pp).

Roitt I.M. *Essential Immunology*, 4th edn. Blackwell Scientific Publications, Oxford, 1980 (374 pp).

Thaler, M.S., Klausner R.D. & Cohen, H.J. *Medical Immunology*. J.B. Lippincott Co., Philadelphia, 1977 (480 pp).

Weir D.M. *Immunology*. Churchill Livingstone, Edinburgh, 1977 (206 pp).

List of figures

1 The scope of immunology

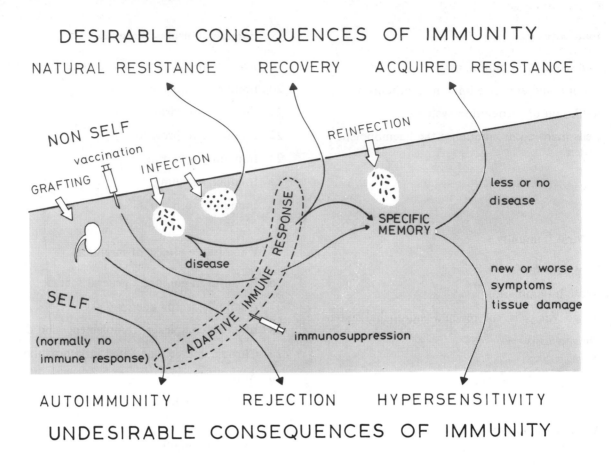

DESIRABLE CONSEQUENCES OF IMMUNITY

NATURAL RESISTANCE   RECOVERY   ACQUIRED RESISTANCE

NON SELF

vaccination

GRAFTING   INFECTION

REINFECTION

disease

SELF

ADAPTIVE IMMUNE RESPONSE

SPECIFIC MEMORY

less or no disease

new or worse symptoms tissue damage

(normally no immune response)

immunosuppression

AUTOIMMUNITY   REJECTION   HYPERSENSITIVITY

UNDESIRABLE CONSEQUENCES OF IMMUNITY

Immunity is concerned with the recognition and disposal of foreign or 'non-self' material that enters the body (white arrows in the figure), whether in the form of life-threatening infectious micro-organisms or a life-saving kidney graft. Resistance to infection may be **'natural'** (i.e. inborn and unchanging) or **'acquired'** as the result of an **adaptive immune response** (centre).

Immunology is the study of the organs, cells, and molecules responsible for this recognition and disposal (the 'immune system'), of how they respond and interact, of the consequences — desirable (top) or otherwise (bottom) — of their activity, and of the ways in which they can be advantageously increased or reduced.

Note that some scientists (e.g. Soviet) extend immunology to include other relationships between cells, for instance during embryonic development, at which most Western immunologists draw the line. Nature, presumably, is not prejudiced as to which type of specialist unveils her secrets, but the more restricted approach does so far seem to have led to more rapid progress. However it is hard to imagine that in the long run immunologists and embryologists will not join forces, **recognition** being central to both disciplines.

Non-self

A term covering everything which is detectably different from an animal's own constituents. Micro-organisms, together with cells, organs, or other materials from another animal, are the most important non-self substances from an immunological viewpoint, but drugs and even normal foods can sometimes give rise to immunity.

Infection

Viruses, bacteria, protozoa, worms, or fungi that attempt to gain access to the body or its surfaces are probably the chief *raison d'être* of the immune system.

Natural resistance

Entry of many micro-organisms (shown in the figure as black dots) is prevented, or they are rapidly eliminated, by antimicrobial defence mechanisms. Others (shown as black rods) can survive to cause disease.

Adaptive immune response

The development or augmentation of defence mechanisms in response to a particular ('specific') stimulus. It can result in elimination of the micro-organism and **recovery** from disease, and often leaves the host with **specific memory**, enabling it to respond more effectively on reinfection with the same micro-organism, a condition called **acquired resistance.**

Vaccination

A method of stimulating the adaptive immune response and generating memory and acquired resistance without suffering disease.

Grafting

Cells or organs from another individual usually survive natural resistance mechanisms but are attacked by the adaptive immune response, leading to **rejection**.

Autoimmunity

The body's own ('self') cells and molecules do not normally stimulate its adaptive immune responses for various reasons covered by the term 'self-tolerance', but in certain circumstances they do and the body's own structures are attacked as if they were foreign, a condition called **autoimmunity** or **autoimmune disease**.

Hypersensitivity

Sometimes the result of specific memory is that re-exposure to the same stimulus, as well as or instead of eliminating the stimulus, has unpleasant or damaging effects on the body's own tissues. This is called **hypersensitivity**; examples are allergy (i.e. hay fever) and some forms of kidney disease. (Note however that the term 'allergy' is used by some immunologists to describe *all* alterations in responsiveness, in which case it also includes acquired resistance).

Immunosuppression

Autoimmunity, hypersensititivty, and particularly graft rejection, sometimes necessitate the suppression of adaptive immune responses by drugs or other means.

2 Natural and adaptive immune mechanisms

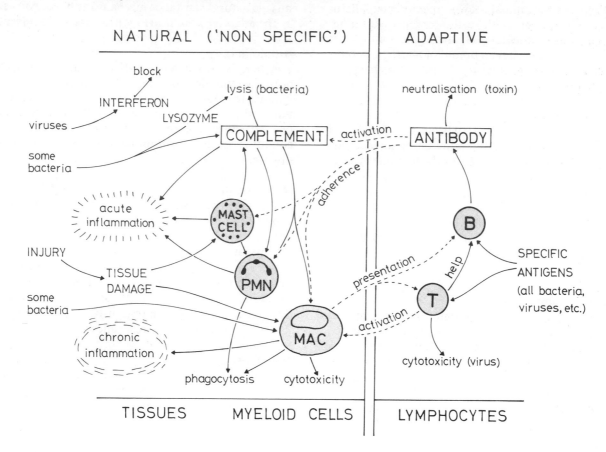

Just as resistance to disease can be natural or acquired, the mechanisms mediating it can be correspondingly divided into **natural** (left) and **adaptive** (right), each composed of both **cellular** (shaded) and **humoral** (i.e. free in serum or body fluids; upper half) elements. Adaptive mechanisms, more recently evolved, perform many of their functions by interacting with the older natural ones.

The mechanisms involved in natural immunity are largely the same as those responsible for non-specifically reacting to tissue damage with the production of **inflammation**, (cover up the right-hand part of the figure to appreciate this). However some cells (e.g. macrophages) and humoral factors (complement, lysozyme) do also have a limited ability to recognise and dispose of bacteria, while most cells can secrete the antiviral agent interferon. Thus the term 'non-specific', though often used as a synonym for 'natural', is not completely accurate.

Adaptive immunity is based on the special properties of **lymphocytes** (T and B, lower right), which can respond selectively to thousands of different non-self materials, or 'antigens', leading to specific memory and a permanently altered pattern of response — an *adaptation* to the animal's own environment. Adaptive mechanisms can function on their own against certain antigens (cover up the left-hand part of the figure), but the majority of their effects are exerted by means of the interaction of antibody with complement and the phagocytic cells of natural immunity, and of T cells with macrophages (broken lines). Through their activation of these natural mechanisms, adaptive responses frequently provoke inflammation, either acute or chronic; when it becomes a nuisance this is called **hypersensitivity**.

The individual elements of this highly simplified scheme are illustrated in more detail in the remainder of this book.

NATURAL IMMUNITY

Interferon A family of proteins produced rapidly by many cells in response to virus infection, which block the replication of virus in other cells.

Lysozyme (Muramidase) An enzyme secreted by macrophages, which attacks the cell wall of some bacteria. Interferon and lysozyme are sometimes described as 'natural antibiotics'.

Complement A series of enzymes present in serum which when activated produce widespread inflammatory effects, as well as lysis of bacteria, etc. Some bacteria activate complement directly, while others only do so with the help of antibody.

Lysis Irreversible leakage of cell contents following membrane damage.

Mast cell A large tissue cell which releases inflammatory mediators when damaged, and also under the influence of antibody. By increasing vascular permeability, inflammation allows complement and cells to enter the tissues from the blood.

PMN polymorphonuclear leucocyte, a short-lived 'scavenger' blood cell, whose granules contain powerful bactericidal enzymes.

MAC macrophage, a large tissue cell responsible for removing damaged tissue, cells, bacteria, etc. Both PMN's and macrophages come from bone marrow, and are therefore known as **myeloid** cells.

Phagocytosis ('cell eating') Engulfment of a particle by a cell. Macrophages and PMN's (which used to be called 'microphages') are the most important phagocytic cells.

Cytotoxicity Macrophages can kill some targets (perhaps including tumour cells) without phagocytosing them.

ADAPTIVE IMMUNITY

Antigen Strictly speaking, a substance which stimulates the production of **antibody**. The term is often applied, however, to substances that stimulate any type of adaptive immune response. Typically, antigens are foreign ('non-self') and either particulate (e.g. cells, bacteria etc) or large protein or polysaccharide molecules. But under special conditions small molecules and even 'self' components can become antigenic.

Specific; specificity Terms used to denote the production of an immune response more or less selective for the stimulus, e.g. a lymphocyte that responds to, or an antibody that 'fits', a particular antigen.

Lymphocyte A small cell found in blood, from which it recirculates through the tissues and back via the lymph, 'policing' the body for non-self material. Its ability to recognise individual antigens through its specialised surface receptors and to divide into numerous cells of identical specificity and long life-span, makes it the ideal cell for adaptive responses. Two major populations of lymphocytes are recognised: T and B.

B lymphocytes secrete antibody, the humoral element of adaptive immunity.

T ('thymus-derived') lymphocytes are further divided into subpopulations which 'help' B lymphocytes, kill virus-infected cells, activate macrophages, etc.

Antibody Serum globulins with a wide range of specificity for different antigens. Antibodies can bind to and neutralise bacterial toxins, and also, by binding to the surface of bacteria, viruses, or other parasites, increase their adherence to, and phagocytosis by, myeloid cells. This can be even further increased by the ability of many antibodies to activate complement.

Presentation of antigens to T and B cells by special macrophages is necessary for most adaptive responses; this is an example of 'reverse interaction' between adaptive and natural immune mechanisms.

Help by T cells is required for the secretion of most antibodies by B cells. There are also 'suppressor' T cells which have the opposite effect.

3 Evolution of recognition systems

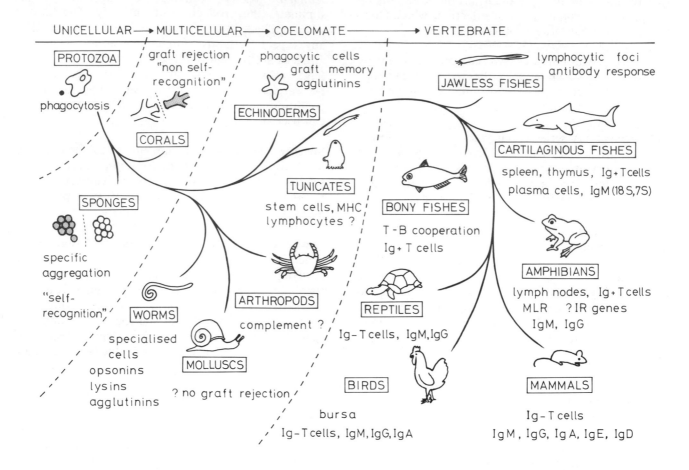

From the humble amoeba searching for food (top left) to the mammal with its sophisticated humoral and cellular immune mechanisms (bottom right), the process of **'self versus non-self recognition'** shows a steady development, keeping pace with the increasing need of animals to maintain their integrity in a hostile environment. The decision at which point 'immunity' appeared is thus a purely semantic one.

In this figure are shown some of the important landmarks in this development. Since most advances, once achieved, persist in subsequent species, they have for clarity been shown only where they are first thought to have appeared. It must be remembered that our knowledge of primitive animals is based largely on study of their modern descendants, all of whom evidently have immune systems adequate to their circumstances.

In so far as the T cell system is based on the cellular recognition of 'altered-self' or 'not-quite-self', it appears to have its roots considerably further back in evolution than antibody, which is roughly restricted to vertebrates.

Protozoa Lacking chlorophyll, these little animals must eat. Little is known about how they recognise 'food', but their surface proteins are under quite complex genetic control.

Sponges Partly free-living, partly colonial, sponge cells use species-specific glycoproteins to identify 'self' and prevent hybrid colony formation.

Corals Corals accept genetically identical grafts (syngrafts) but slowly reject non-identical ones (allografts) with damage to both partners. There is some evidence for specific memory of a previous rejection — i.e. of 'adaptive' immunity.

Worms A feature of all coelomate animals is cell specialisation. In the earthworm coelom there are at least four cell types, some of which are involved in allograft rejection, while others may produce antibacterial factors; all are phagocytic.

Molluscs and **Arthropods** are curious in apparently not showing graft rejection. However humoral factors are prominent, possibly including the earliest complement components.

Echinoderms The starfish is famous for Metchnikoff's classic demonstration of specialised phagocytic cells (1882). Allografts are rejected, with cellular infiltration, and there is a strong specific memory response.

Tunicates (e.g. Amphioxus, sea-squirts) These pre-vertebrates show several advanced features; self-renewing haemopoietic cells, lymphoid-like cells, and a single major histocompatibility complex (MHC) controlling allograft rejection.

Jawless fishes (cyclostomes, e.g. hagfish, lamprey) The earliest surviving vertebrates, with lymphoid cells organised into foci in the pharynx and elsewhere, and the first definite antibody immunoglobulin (Ig), a labile four-chain molecule, produced specifically in response to a variety of antigens: a dramatic moment in the evolution of the immune system.

Cartilaginous fishes (e.g. sharks) The first appearance of the thymus, of the secondary antibody response, and of plasma cells (specialised for high-rate antibody secretion) marks another tremendous step. Ig chains are now disulphide-linked; the high and low molecular weight forms probably represent polymerisation rather than class differences.

Bony fish The different responses to mitogens and the evidence for cell cooperation in antibody production suggest that T and B lymphocyte functions have begun to separate.

Amphibians The first appearance of another Ig class (IgG) and of the mixed-lymphocyte reaction (MLR). An important new region (I region) may have been added to the MHC at this stage.

Reptiles It is interesting that fish and amphibian thymus cells carry Ig similar to that in serum, while in reptiles, birds, and mammals they carry either no Ig or a molecule which is part-Ig, part MHC-product.

Birds are unusual in producing their B lymphocytes exclusively in a special organ, the Bursa of Fabricius, near the cloaca.

Mammals are characterised more by Ig class and subclass diversity than by any further development of T-cell functions.

4 Cells involved in immunity: the haemopoietic system

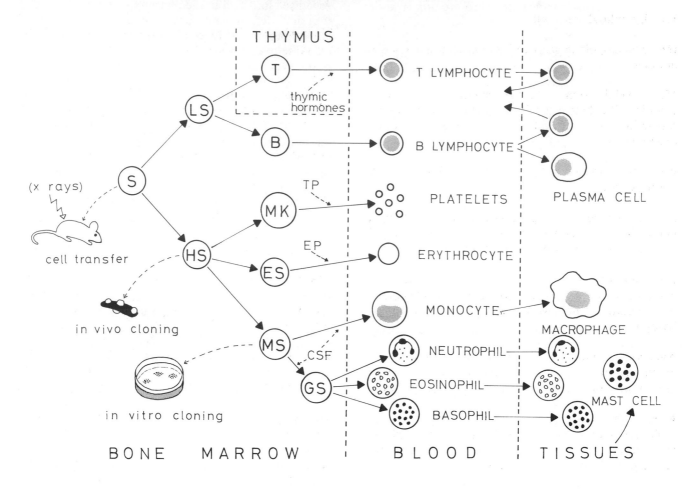

The great majority of cells involved in mammalian immunity are derived from precursors in the bone marrow (left half of figure) and circulate in the blood, entering and sometimes leaving the tissues when required.

The existence of the long-debated totipotent **stem cell** in the adult, retaining the 'embryonic' ability to differentiate into all types of blood cell, has been established by cell-transfer experiments and chromosome analysis in irradiated mice (centre left); stem cells are probably restricted to the bone marrow, and very rare there (about 1 in 10^5 cells). By injecting small numbers of marrow cells, discrete spleen nodules, or '*in vivo* clones' can be grown, whose morphology and differentiation can be studied in a more or less natural environment. Similar experiments in semi-solid culture conditions *in vitro* enable the clonal progeny of single marrow cells to be examined in complete isolation (lower left).

Unlike other haemopoietic cells, lymphocytes do not normally divide unless stimulated, and the propagation of lymphocyte clones usually requires repeated exposure to antigen, followed by selection of specifically reactive cells. But a promising development is the fusion of specific T or B lymphocytes with a tumour cell, to produce an immortal hybrid clone or 'hybridoma', of great value in studying the properties of lymphocytes, which are complex and varied (see Fig 9).

A note on terminology
Haematologists recognise many stages between stem cells and their fully differentiated progeny (e.g. for the red cells: proerythroblast; erythroblast, normoblast, erythrocyte). The suffix-**blast** usually implies an early, dividing, relatively undifferentiated cell, but is also used to describe lymphocytes that have been stimulated, e.g. by antigen, and are about to divide; whence 'blast transformation'.

S Stem cell; the totipotent marrow cell, of proved existence but uncertain morphology.

LS Lymphoid stem cell.

HS Haemopoietic stem cell; the precursor of spleen nodules.

MS Myeloid stem cell; the precursor of *in vitro* colonies. The three last cells are assumed to have some restriction of potential on the basis of cloning experiments.

ES Erythroid stem cell, destined to differentiate into erythrocytes.

EP Erythropoieten; a glycoprotein hormone formed in the kidney in response to hypoxia, which accelerates the differentiation of erythrocyte precursors.

GS Granulocyte stem cell; a cell presumed to be committed to granulocyte production but capable of differentiation into either neutrophil, eosinophil, or basophil leucocytes.

Neutrophil (polymorph) The commonest leucocyte of the blood, a short-lived phagocytic cell whose granules contain numerous bactericidal substances.

Eosinophil A leucocyte with large refractile eosinophilic granules, phagocytic and perhaps cytotoxic for some larger parasites, such as worms. It may also regulate the inflammatory response.

Basophil A leucocyte whose large basophilic granules contain heparin and vasoactive amines, important in the inflammatory response.

Monocyte The largest nucleated cell of the blood, developing into a macrophage when it migrates into the tissues.

Macrophage The principal resident phagocyte of the tissues and serous cavities.

CSF Colony stimulating factor(s); substances produced by various kinds of cell, required for the development of *in vitro* clones. There are also inhibitory factors, possibly including interferon.

MK Megakaryocyte; the parent cell of the blood platelets.

TP Thrombopoietin; a hormone that regulates the production of platelets.

T Thymus-derived (or -processed) lymphocyte.

Thymic hormones Numerous small peptides extracted from thymic epithelium (e.g. 'thymosin') are thought by some to assist the differentiation of T lymphocytes.

B Bone marrow- (or, in birds, Bursa-) derived lymphocyte, the precursor of antibody-forming cells. In foetal life, the liver may play the role of 'Bursa'.

Plasma cell A B cell in its high-rate antibody secreting state.

Mast cell A large tissue cell similar in appearance and function to the basophil, but thought not to originate from the bone marrow. Mast cells are easily triggered by tissue damage to initiate the inflammatory response.

5 Complement

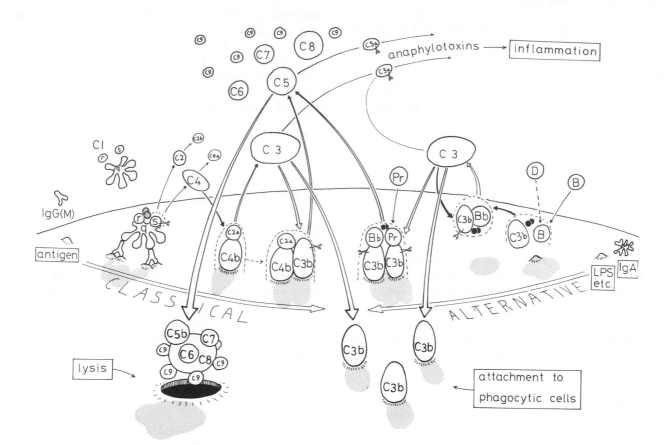

Fifteen or more serum components constitute the **complement** system, the sequential activation and assembly into functional units of which leads to three main effects: release of peptides active in **inflammation** (top right), deposition of C3b, a powerful attachment-promoter (or 'opsonin') for **phagocytosis**, on cell membranes (bottom right), and membrane damage resulting in **lysis** (bottom left). Together these make it an important part of the defences against micro-organisms. Defects of some components can predispose to severe infections, particularly bacterial.

The upper half of the figure represents the serum, or 'fluid' phase, the lower half the cell surface, where activation (indicated by dotted haloes) and assembly

largely occur. Activation of complement can proceed by two distinct routes, the **'classical'** (because first described) pathway, initiated by the binding of specific antibody of the IgG or IgM class (see Fig 12) to surface antigens (centre left), and the **'alternative'**, but probably more primitive, pathway, initiated by a variety of polysaccharides and by aggregates of IgA (centre right). Some of the steps are dependent on the divalent ions Ca^{2+} (shaded circles) or Mg^{2+} (black circles).

Activation is usually limited to the immediate vicinity by the very short life of the active products, and in some cases there are special inactivators (χ). Nevertheless, excessive complement activation can cause unpleasant side-effects (see Fig 28).

CLASSICAL PATHWAY

For many years this was the only way in which complement was known to be activated. The essential feature is the requirement for a specific antigen – antibody interaction, leading via components C1, C2 and C4 to the formation of a 'convertase' which splits C3.

Ig IgM and some subclasses of IgG (in the human, IgG3,1, and 2), when bound to antigen are recognized by Clq to initiate the classical pathway.

C1 A Ca^{2+} dependent union of three components: Clq (MW 400,000), a curious protein with six valencies for Ig linked by collagen-like fibrils, which activates in turn Clr (MW 170,000) and Cls (MW 80,000), a serine esterase which goes on to attack C2 and C4.

C2 (MW 120,000), split by Cls into small (C2b) and large (C2a) fragments.

C4 (MW 240,000), likewise split into C4a (small) and C4b (large). C4b and C2a then join together and attach to the antigen – antibody complex, or to the membrane in the case of a cell-bound antigen, forming a 'C3 convertase'.

C3 (MW 180,000), the central component of all complement reactions, split by its convertase into a small (C3a) and a large fragment (C3b). Some of the C3b is deposited on the membrane, where it serves as an attachment site for phagocytic polymorphs and macrophages, which have receptors for it; some remains associated with C2a and C4b, forming a 'C5 convertase'. An enzyme, 'C3b inactivator' or KAF rapidly inactivates C3b, releasing the fragment C3c and leaving membrane-bound C3d.

C5 (MW 180,000), split by its convertase into C5a, a small peptide which, together with C3a (anaphylotoxins), acts on mast cells, polymorphs, and smooth muscle to promote the inflammatory response, and C5b, which initiates the assembly of C6, 7, 8 and 9 into the membrane-damaging or 'lytic' unit.

ALTERNATIVE PATHWAY

The principal features distinguishing this from the classical pathway are the lack of dependence on calcium ions and the lack of need for C1, C2, or C4, and therefore for specific antigen – antibody interaction. Instead, several different molecules can initiate C3 conversion, notably lipopolysaccharides and other bacterial products, but also including aggregates of some types of antibody such as IgA. Essentially the alternative pathway consists of a continuously 'ticking over' cycle, held in check by control molecules whose effects are counteracted by the various initiators.

B Factor B (MW 100,000), which complexes with C3b, whether produced via the classical pathway or the alternative pathway itself. It has both structural and functional similarities to C2, and both are coded for by genes within the very important Major Histocompatibility Complex (see Fig 17).

D Factor D (MW 25,000), an enzyme which acts on the C3b-B complex to produce the active convertase.

Pr Properdin (MW 220,000), the first isolated component of the alternative pathway, once thought to be the actual initiator but now known merely to stabilise the C3b-B complex so that it can act on further C3. Thus more C3b is produced which, with Factors B and D, leads in turn to further C3 conversion — a 'positive feedback' loop with great amplifying potential (but restrained by the C3b inactivator KAF).

LYTIC PATHWAY

Lysis of cells is probably the least vital of the complement reactions, but one of the easiest to study. It is initiated by the splitting of C5 by one of its two convertases: C3b-C2a-C4b (classical pathway) or C3b-B-Pr (alternative pathway). Thereafter the results are the same however caused.

C6 (MW 150,000), **C7** (MW 140,000) and **C8** (MW 150,000) unite with C5b, one molecule of each, and with six molecules of **C9** (MW 80,000). Membrane damage was once thought to be due to a phospholipase activity of this complex but now looks more like an ionophore ('channel') effect. Red cells are lysed, but some bacteria require the action of lysozyme as well for complete lysis.

6 Acute inflammation

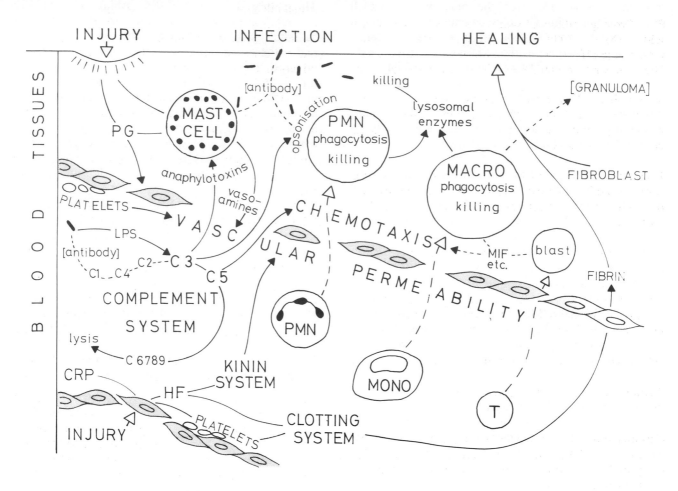

Whether **inflammation** should be considered part of immunology is a problem for the teaching profession, not for the body — which combats infection by all the means at its disposal, including mechanisms also involved in the response to and repair of other types of damage.

In this simplified scheme are shown the effects of **injury** to tissues (top left) and to blood vessels (bottom left). The small black rods represent bacterial **infection**, a very common cause of inflammation. Note the central role of permeability of the vascular endothelium (shaded) in allowing access of blood cells

and serum components (lower half) to the tissues (upper half), which also accounts for the main symptoms of inflammation — redness, warmth, swelling, and pain.

It can be seen that the 'adaptive' (or 'immunological') functions of antibody and lymphocytes largely operate to amplify or focus pre-existing 'natural' mechanisms; quantitatively, however, they are so important that they frequently make the difference between life and death. Further details of the role of antibody and lymphocytes in inflammation will be found in Figs 26-29.

Mast cell A large tissue cell with basophilic granules containing vasoactive amines and heparin.

PG Prostaglandins; a family of unsaturated fatty acids (MW 300 – 400) with stimulatory and suppressive effects on many inflammatory processes. They appear to be made principally by macrophages.

Vasoamines Vasoactive amines; e.g. histamine, 5-hydroxytryptamine, produced by mast cells, basophils, and platelets, and causing increased capillary permeability.

Complement A cascading sequence of serum proteins, activated either directly ('alternate pathway') or via antigen-antibody interaction ('classical pathway').

C142 The classical pathway, activated by antibody if present.

C3 The most abundant and important component, producing when activated a small (C3a) and a large peptide (C3b).

C5 Similarly split (by C3b) into C5a and C5b.

Anaphylotoxins C3a and C5a, which stimulate release by mast cells of their vasoactive amines.

Opsonisation C3b attached to a particle promotes sticking to phagocytic cells because of their 'C3 receptors'. Antibody, if present, augments this by binding to 'Fc receptors'.

C6789 The lytic pathway, activated by C5b and culminating in puncture of cell membranes.

LPS Lipopolysaccharide; the major component of bacterial cell walls, which protects them from phagocytosis but activates C3 directly.

CRP C-reactive protein (MW 130,000), a globulin which appears in the serum within hours of tissue damage or infection. It may play an antibody-like role in opsonising some bacteria. Proteins whose serum concentration increases during inflammation are called 'acute phase proteins'; they include CRP and many complement components.

Kinin system A series of serum peptides sequentially activated to cause vasodilatation and increased permeability.

Clotting system Intimately bound up with complement and kinins because of several shared activation steps.

HF Hageman factor ('clotting factor XII'), the common trigger for the kinin and clotting (and fibrinolytic) systems.

Fibrin the end product of blood clotting and, in the tissues, the matrix into which fibroblasts migrate to initiate healing.

PMN Polymorphonuclear leucocyte.

Mono Monocyte; the precursor of tissue macrophages.

Lysosomal enzymes Bactericidal enzymes released from the lysosomes of PMN's, monocytes, and macrophages, e.g. lysozyme, myeloperoxidase.

T T lymphocyte, undergoing **blast** transformation if stimulated by antigen.

Chemotaxis C5a, C3a, and some lymphocyte products stimulate PMN's and monocytes to move into the tissues. Movement towards the site of inflammation is called chemotaxis, and is presumably due to the cells' ability to detect a concentration gradient of chemotactic factors; random increases of movement are called chemokinesis.

MIF Macrophage migration inhibitory factor; a lymphocyte product chemotactic for monocytes. Other similar factors stimulate monocyte and macrophage functions.

Granuloma A macrophage-derived lesion in which are sequestered noxious agents (foreign bodies, some bacteria, etc) which cannot be eliminated.

7 Phagocytic cells: the reticulo-endothelial system

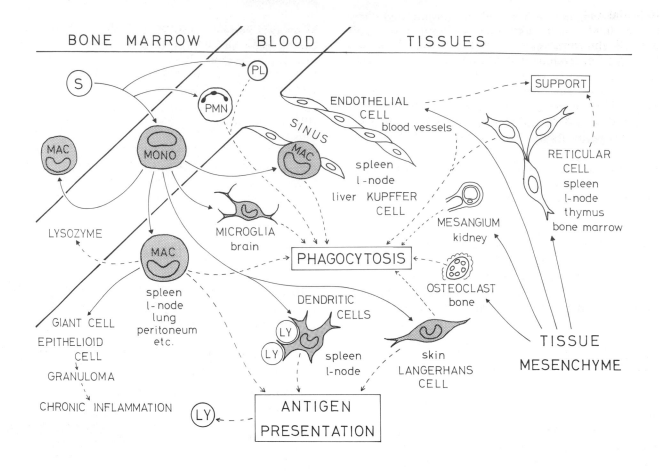

Particulate matter which finds its way into the blood or tissues is rapidly removed by cells, and the property of taking up dyes, colloids, etc, was used by anatomists to define a body-wide system of phagocytic cells known as the **'reticulo-endothelial system'** (RES), consisting of the vascular endothelium and reticular tissue cells (top right), and — supposedly descended from these — various types of macrophages whose routine functons included clearing up the body's own debris, and killing and digesting bacteria.

However more modern work has shown a fundamental distinction between those phagocytic cells derived from the bone marrow via the blood monocyte (shaded) and others formed locally from the tissues themselves (right side of figure). Ironically, neither reticular nor endothelial cells are outstandingly phagocytic, their function being mainly structural.

More recently still, attention has focussed on the interactions between the RES and adaptive immunity. The role of antibody in amplifying phagocytosis and of T lymphocytes in activating other macrophage functions, is discussed in Figs 8 and 29, but it is worth noting here that neither B nor T lymphocytes can normally respond to foreign antigens unless the latter are properly **'presented'**. It used to be assumed that the presenting cells were typical macrophages, but there is growing evidence that there are special separate populations of cells in the skin and the lymphoid organs (lower centre) with the ability to bind antigens and to interact with lymphocytes. When this process is fully understood, there may be some hope of a rational classification of this whole group of cells.

Endothelial cell The inner lining of blood vessels, able to take up dyes etc, but not truly phagocytic.

Reticular cell The main supporting or 'stromal' cell of lymphoid organs, usually associated with collagen-like reticulin fibres, and not easily distinguished from fibroblasts or from other branching or 'dendritic' cells (see below) — whence a great deal of confusion.

Mesangium Mesangial cells give support to the glomerulus, and may phagocytose material deposited in it, particularly complexes of antigen and antibody.

Osteoclast A large multinucleate cell responsible for resorbing and so shaping bone. There is some evidence that its function can be regulated by T lymphocytes.

Dendritic cells The weakly phagocyte **Langerhans cell** of the epidermis, and somewhat similar but non-phagocytic cells in the lymphoid follicles of the spleen and lymph nodes, may be the main agent of T-cell stimulation; T cells recognise foreign antigens in association with cell-surface antigens (collectively known as **Ia**) coded for by the Major Histocompatibility Complex, a genetic region intimately involved in immune responses of all kinds (see Fig 17). There are probably separate dendritic cells for presenting antigen to B cells. All cells of this type appear to be derived ultimately from the bone marrow.

Ly Lymphocytes are often found in close contact with dendritic cells; this is presumably where antigen presentation and T-B cell cooperation take place.

S The totipotent bone marrow stem cell, giving rise to all the cells found in blood.

PL Blood platelets, though primarily involved in clotting, are able to phagocytose antigen-antibody complexes.

PMN Polymorphonuclear leucocyte, the major phagocytic cell of the blood, not, however, conventionally considered as part of the RES.

Mono Monocyte, formed in the narrow and travelling via the blood to the tissues, where it matures into a macrophage. It is likely, though not proved, that the specialised antigen-presenting cells also develop from monocytes.

Mac Macrophage, the resident and long-lived tissue phagocyte. Macrophages may be either free in the tissues, or 'fixed' in the walls of blood sinuses, where they monitor the blood for particles, effete red cells, etc. This activity is strongest in the liver, where the macrophages are called Kupffer cells. Macrophages (and polymorphs) have the valuable ability to recognise not only foreign matter but also antibody and/or complement bound to it, which greatly enhances phagocytosis (see Fig 8).

Sinus Tortuous channels in liver, spleen etc, through which blood passes to reach the veins, allowing the lining macrophages to remove damaged or antibody-coated cells.

Microglia The phagocytic cells of the brain, thought to be derived from incoming blood monocytes.

Lysozyme An important anti-bacterial enzyme secreted into the blood by macrophages. Macrophages also produce other 'natural' humoral factors such as interferon and many complement components.

Giant cell; epithelioid cell Macrophage-derived cells typically found at sites of chronic inflammation; by coalescing into a solid mass, or **granuloma**, they localise and wall off irritant or indigestible materials.

8 Phagocytosis

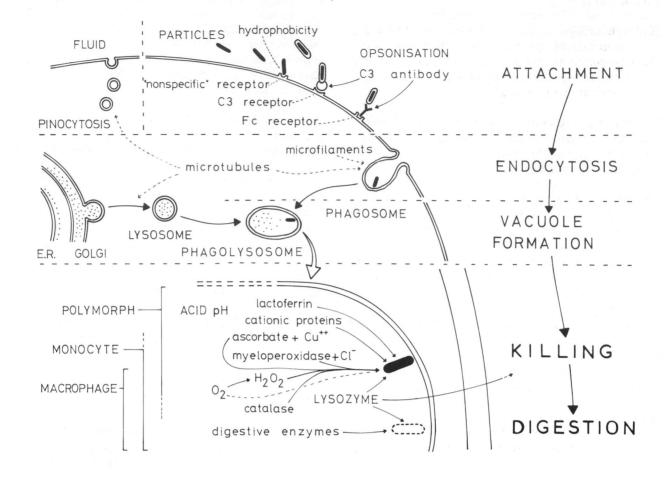

Numerous cells are able to ingest foreign materials, but the ability to increase this activity in response to opsonisation by antibody and/or complement, so as to acquire antigen-specificity, is restricted to cells of the myeloid series, principally the **polymorphs, monocytes**, and **macrophages**; these are sometimes termed 'professional' phagocytes.

Apart from some variations in their content of lysosomal enzymes, all myeloid cells use essentially similar mechanisms to phagocytose foreign objects, consisting of a sequence of **attachment** (top), endocytosis or **ingestion** (centre), and **digestion** (bottom). In the figure this process is shown for a typical bacterium (small black rods). In general, bacteria with **capsules** (shown outlined) are not phagocytosed unless opsonised, whereas many non-capsulated ones do not require this. There are certain differences between phagocytic cells, for example polymorphs are very short-lived (hours or days) and often die in the process of phagocytosis, whilst macrophages, which lack some of the more destructive enzymes, usually survive to phagocytose again. Also macrophages can actively secrete some of their enzymes, e.g. lysozyme. There are surprisingly large species differences in the proportions of the various lysosomal enzymes.

Several of the steps in phagocytosis shown in the figure may be specifically defective for genetic reasons (see Fig 33), as well as being actively inhibited by particular micro-organisms (see Figs 20, 22, 24). In either case the result is a failure to eliminate micro-organisms or foreign material properly, leading to chronic infection and/or chronic inflammation.

Pinocytosis 'Cell drinking'; the ingestion of soluble materials, conventionally applied to particles under 1μm in diameter.

Hydrophobicity Hydrophobic groups tend to attach to the hydrophobic surface of cells; this may explain the 'recognition' of damaged cells, denatured proteins, etc. Bacterial capsules, largely polysaccharide, reduce hydrophobicity and block attachment.

Non-specific receptor Another view is that phagocytic cells have surface structures complementary to the wide range of materials they recognise and attach to.

C3 receptor Phagocytic cells (and some lymphocytes) can bind C3b, produced from C3 by activation by bacteria etc, either directly or via antibody.

Fc receptor Phagocytic cells (and most lymphocytes, platelets, etc) can bind the Fc portion of antibody, especially of the IgG class.

Opsonisation refers to the promotion or enhancement of attachment via the C3 or Fc receptor.

Phagosome A vacuole formed by the internalisation of surface membrane along with an attached particle.

Microtubules Short rigid structures that arrange themselves into channels for vacuoles etc. to travel within the cell, and also serve to stiffen the membrane.

Microfilaments Contractile protein (actin) filaments responsible for membrane activities such as pinocytosis and phagosome formation.

E.R. Endoplasmic reticulum; a membranous system of sacs and tubules with which ribosomes are associated in the synthesis of many proteins for secretion.

Golgi The region where products of the ER are packaged into vesicles.

Lysosome A membrane-bound package of hydrolytic enzymes usually active at acid pH (e.g. acid phosphatase, DNA-ase). Lysosomes are found in almost all cells, and are vehicles for secretion as well as digestion. They are prominent in macrophages and polymorphs, which also have separate vesicles containing lysozyme and other enzymes; together with lysosomes these constitute the **granules** whose staining patterns characterise the various types of polymorph (neutrophil, basophil, eosinophil). Newly formed lysosomes not containing any substrate are sometimes called 'primary'.

Phagolysosome A vacuole formed by the fusion of a phagosome and lysosome(s), in which micro-organisms are killed and digested.

Lactoferrin A protein that inhibits bacteria by depriving them of iron.

Cationic proteins Examples are 'phagocytin', 'leukin'; microbicidal agents found in some polymorph granules.

Ascorbate interacts with copper ions and hydrogen peroxide, and can be bactericidal.

Myeloperoxidase An important microbicidal enzyme in conjunction with hydrogen peroxide and halide (e.g. chloride) ions. It is absent from mature macrophages but may be partly replaced by catalase.

O_2, H_2O_2 Free radicals such as O_2 and OH may be bactericidal as well as giving rise to hydrogen peroxide.

Lysozyme (muramidase) lyses many saprophytes (e.g. M. lysodeicticus) and some pathogenic bacteria damaged by antibody and/or complement. It is a major secretory product of macrophages.

Digestive enzymes The enzymes by which lysosomes are usually identified, such as acid phosphatase, lipase, elastase, β glucuronidase, etc.

9 Lymphocytes

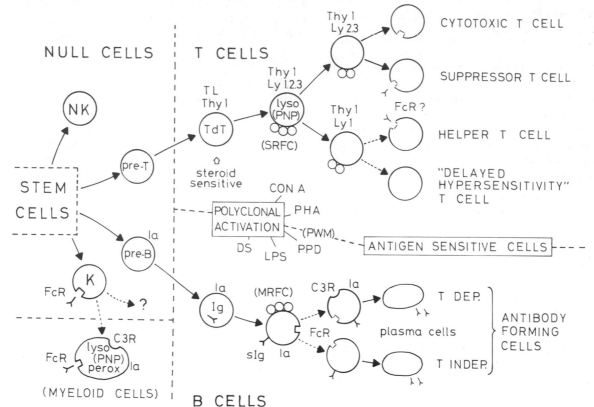

NULL CELLS | T CELLS

NK

STEM CELLS

pre-T

pre-B

FcR — K — ?

la Ig

FcR lyso (PNP) perox la C3R

(MYELOID CELLS)

B CELLS

TL Thy1 TdT

↑ steroid sensitive

Thy1 Ly 1.2.3 lyso (PNP) (SRFC)

Thy 1 Ly 2.3

Thy 1 Ly 1

CYTOTOXIC T CELL

SUPPRESSOR T CELL

FcR ?

HELPER T CELL

"DELAYED HYPERSENSITIVITY" T CELL

CON A

POLYCLONAL ACTIVATION

PHA

(PWM)

DS LPS PPD

ANTIGEN SENSITIVE CELLS

la (MRFC) C3R la

sIg la

FcR

plasma cells

T DEP.

T INDEP.

ANTIBODY FORMING CELLS

As befits the cell of adaptive immunity, the lymphocyte has several unique features: restricted receptors permitting each cell to respond to an individual antigen (the basis of **specificity**), clonal proliferation and long lifespan (the basis of **memory**), and recirculation from the tissues back into the bloodstream, which ensures that specific memory following a local response has a bodywide **distribution**.

The discovery of the two major lymphocyte sub-populations, **T** (thymus-dependent; top) and **B** (Bursa or bone marrow dependent; bottom), had roughly the same impact on cellular immunology as the double helix on molecular biology. The first property of T cells to be distinguished was that of 'helping' B cells to make antibody, but further subdivisions have subsequently come to light, based on both functional and physical differences; four types of T cell are now recognised (top right). In the figure, the main surface features (or 'markers') of the various stages of lymphocyte differentiation are given for the mouse, with some special markers of human subpopulations shown in brackets. The latter have been of particular value in classifying lymphoid and myeloid malignancies (leukaemia).

Cells resembling lymphocytes, but without characteristic T or B cell markers are referred to as

'null' (left). This group probably includes early T cells, B cells, and monocytes, as well as the 'natural killer' cells possibly important in tumour imunity. In blood and lymphoid organs, up to 10% of lymphocytes are 'null'.

In one of the most exciting recent developments in biology, it has been found possible to perpetuate individual lymphocytes by fusing them with a tumour cell. In the case of B lymphocytes, this can mean an endless supply of individual, or **monoclonal**, antibodies, with far-reaching applications in the diagnosis and treatment of disease and the study of cell surfaces. Indeed, it is likely that the classification of lymphocytes themselves, and of most other cells too, will soon be based on patterns of reactivity with a large range of monoclonal typing antisera.

NULL CELLS

NK Natural killer cell, cytotoxic to some tumours, apparently in the absence of antibody. Its lineage is unknown.

K The 'killer' lymphocyte of antibody-dependent cytotoxicity (ADCC) *in vitro*, of unproved *in vivo* significance.

Myeloid cells Monocytes, macrophages, and granulocytes are also effective in ADCC.

FcR 'Fc receptor'; a receptor for the Fc portion of antibody, especially IgG, which links the ADCC effector cell to its target.

Perox Peroxidase; an important antimicrobial enzyme of monocytes and granulocytes, not found in lymphocytes.

T CELLS

TdT Terminal deoxynucleotidyl transferase, a DNA polymerase found mainly in cortical, and therefore young, thymocytes; these cells are lost from the thymus following corticosteroid treatment.

PNP Purine nucleoside phosphorylase, a purine salvage enzyme, found in human T cells and monocytes, but not B cells; a potentially useful marker.

Lyso Lysosomal enzymes (e.g. acid phosphatase, esterases etc) are found in myeloid cells and to a lesser extent in T cells.

TL Originally 'thymus leukaemia'; a surface antigen of leukaemic and normal mouse thymocytes, absent from mature T cells.

Thy 1 Originally 'theta'; a mouse T-cell surface antigen existing in two allelic forms. It is also found on some brain and skin cells.

Ly 1,2,3 Three separate surface antigens exclusive to T cells (whence the proposed name LyT), each existing in two allelic forms. All are expressed on early T cells, but either 1, or 2 and 3, are largely lost as the cells mature and differentiate. Neither Ly nor Thy 1 molecules themselves have yet been shown to play any part in cell function; however the use of monoclonal antibodies has suggested that a similar system of surface antigens exists on human T cells.

Polyclonal activation Stimulation of a substantial number of lymphocytes, i.e. many clones, rather than the few or single clones normally stimulated by an antigen. Since the first sign of activation is often mitosis, polyclonal activators are sometimes known as 'mitogens'. A surprising number of such 'lectins' are of plant origin and act by a complementary interaction with surface carbohydrates on the cell; this is probably quite fortuitous and has no significance except as a most useful 'marker'.

CON A Concanavalin A (from a bean); stimulates T cells, especially helpers and suppressors, with the production of non-specific helper and suppressor factors.

PHA Phytohaemagglutinin, another T-cell mitogen, probably stimulates a slightly different population of cells from CON A. This was the first mitogen to be discovered, before which lymphocytes were thought to be non-dividing cells!

SRFC Sheep rosette-forming cell; most human T cells bind sheep RBC to make 'rosettes' *in vitro*. The T cells of many species react in the same way with selected heterologous erythrocytes (e.g. cat: guinea-pig). Like the response to mitogens, this is a useful marker without functional significance — which needs to be distinguished from the use of sheep red cells as *antigens*, very common in experimental immunology.

Cytotoxic T cell A key cell in virus immunity. As in all T cell subpopulations, some may express Fc receptors for Ig; it may be (though this is controversial) that whether the receptor is for IgM or IgG is related to the cell's function.

Suppressor T cell Related, and possibly identical to, the above. It can inhibit both B and T-cell responses.

Helper T cell Essential for T-dependent (i.e. most) antibody responses.

Delayed hypersensitivity T cell Important in attracting and activating a variety of cells; helper cells may be a subset of this type.

B CELLS

Ig: sIg Immunoglobulin, at first cytoplasmic and later surface bound, is the key feature of B cells, through which they recognise specific antigens.

Ia Antigens coded by the 'I' region of the Major Histocompatibility Complex, expressed mainly on B cells and macrophages, and involved in the interaction of these with the Ly 1 type of T cells.

C3R 'Complement receptor'; a receptor for split C3 (C3b), found on myeloid cells, where it aids phagocytosis, and on some B cells, chiefly those requiring T-cell help. These cells also express Ia and presumably also a receptor for T-cell derived 'helper factors'.

DS Dextran sulphate.

LPS Lipopolysaccharide, e.g. salmonella endotoxin.

PPD Purified protein derivative (of tuberculin). The above are normally mitogenic only for B cells, possibly at different stages.

PWM Pokeweed mitogen, mitogenic for both T and B cells when both are present. There is unfortunately no ideal mitogen for human B cells.

MRFC Mouse rosette-forming cell; mature human B cells and B cell leukaemias bind mouse erythrocytes *in vitro*.

T dep., T indep. Some antibody formation, especially IgM, does not require T-cell help, and is called 'thymus independent'. It involves different B cells and may be evolutionarily more primitive.

10 Primary lymphoid organs and lymphopoiesis

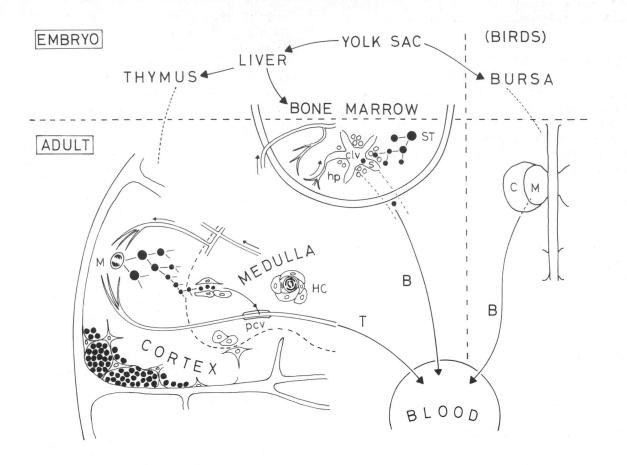

The first strong evidence for distinct lymphocyte populations was the complementary effects in birds of early removal of the **thymus** (which mainly affects cell-mediated immunity) and the **Bursa of Fabricius** (which affects antibody responses). A continuing puzzle has been the identification of what represents the bursa in mammals; despite a phase when 'gut-associated lymphoid tissue' was popular, current opinion considers there to be no true analogue, the liver taking over the function of B cell maturation in the foetus, the bone marrow in the adult.

Another vexed question is why so many cells die in the thymus — up to 90% according to some calculations — and an attractive idea, by no means disproved, is that it is here that self-reactive cells are weeded out. If

the mysterious Hassal's corpuscles turn out to be the site of this process, two enigmas will be resolved at once.

Nor are these the only controversies involving the thymus. The status of its presumed hormones, such as 'thymosin', is still hotly disputed, there are conflicting ideas as to whether all T cells pass from the medulla to the cortex before leaving, or whether a distinct subpopulation leaves directly from the cortex, it is not totally clear what role the thymus plays in determining the pattern of T-cell reactivity to antigens, and finally, despite the lack of solid evidence, many people feel the thymus has something to do with cancer and ageing. (One wonders how long it will be before someone revives Galen's theory that it is the site of the soul!).

YOLK SAC

The source of the earliest haemopoietic tissue, including the lymphocyte precursors.

BURSA

In birds, B lymphocytes differentiate in the Bursa of Fabricus, a cloacal outgrowth with many crypts and follicles, which reaches its maximum size a few weeks after birth and thereafter atrophies. Despite claims for the appendix, tonsil, etc, there is probably no mammalian analogue.

M Medulla; the region where the first stem cells colonise the bursal follicles.

C Cortex; the site of proliferation of the B lymphocytes.

LIVER

During foetal life in mammals, the major haemopoietic and lymphopoietic organ.

BONE MARROW

ST Stem cells for the B cell series.

HP Haemopoietic area. The geographical location of lymphopoiesis in liver and bone marrow is not exactly known, but it presumably proceeds alongside the other haemopoietic pathways.

S Sinus collecting differentiated cells.

CLV Central longitudinal vein, collecting cells from the sinuses for discharge into the blood.

THYMUS

Like the Bursa, the thymus reaches its largest size in early life, though the subsequent atrophy is slower. In the mouse it contains almost exclusively cells of the T series, but in some animals there may be variable numbers of B cells as well. T cell precursors are derived, via the blood, from the bone marrow; they may undergo some degree of differentiation in the marrow under the influence of thymic hormones, but most of their maturation occurs within the thymus itself. Numerous 'soluble factors' extracted from thymus have been shown to stimulate the maturation of T cells, including a nonapeptide of molecular weight less than 1000.

Recent work on the specificity of T cells (see Figs 15 & 16) and the key role of the Major Histocompatibility Complex (see also Fig 17), has suggested that T cells learn first to recognise 'self' antigens, and that this occurs in the thymus. The mechanism is not clear.

Cortex Dark-staining outer part packed with lymphocytes, compartmentalised by elongated epithelial cells.

M Mitotic figures are common; it is thought that about 8 divisions occur between the precursor cell and the exported T cell. Pyknotic nuclei are also common, suggesting that many cells die without leaving the thymus.

Medulla Inner, predominantly epithelial part, to which some (perhaps all) cortical lymphocytes migrate before export.

PCV Post-capillary venule, through which lymphocytes enter the thymic veins and ultimately the blood.

HC Hassal's corpuscle — a structure peculiar to thymus, in which epithelial cells become concentrically compressed and keratinised. It is suspected by some of being the site of production of thymic hormones.

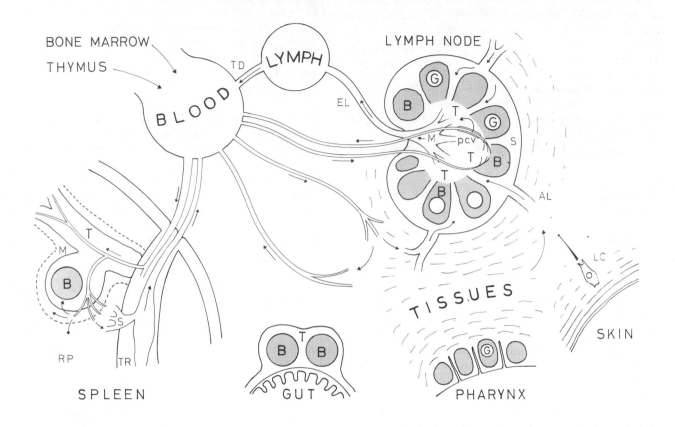

The ability to **recirculate** from blood to tissues and back through the lymphoid system is unique to lymphocytes and, coupled with their long lifespan and specificity for individual antigens, equips them for their central role in adaptive immune responses.

The thorough mixing of lymphocytes, particularly in the **spleen** and **lymph nodes**, ensures the maximum contact of cells that have newly encountered antigen with others potentially able to respond, and the body-wide dissemination of expanded 'memory' populations in readiness for a second encounter with the same antigen.

There is a tendency for different types of lymphocyte to 'home' to different regions in the lymphoid organs (**T** and **B** areas in the figure; **B** areas are shaded). This is presumably due to either chemotactic factors unique to particular sites, or to recognition of different lymphocytes by local elements such as the dendritic antigen-presenting cells (not shown here, but see Fig 7).

In general, lymph nodes respond to antigens introduced into the tissues they drain, and the spleen to antigens in the blood. The gut and external mucous surfaces also have their own less specialised lymphoid organs.

LYMPH NODE

Lymph nodes (or 'glands') constitute the main bulk of the organized lymphoid tissue. They are strategically placed so that lymph from most parts of the body drains through a series of nodes before reaching the Thoracic Duct (**TD**), which empties into the left subclavian vein to allow the lymphocytes to recirculate again via the blood.

AL, EL Afferent and efferent lymphatics, through which lymph passes from the tissues to first peripheral and then central lymph nodes.

S Lymphatic sinus, through which lymph flows from the afferent lymphatic into the cortical and medullary sinuses.

M Medullary sinus, collecting lymph for exit via the efferent lymphatic. It is in the medulla that antibody formation takes place and plasma cells are prominent.

G Germinal centre; an area of larger cells that develops within the follicle after antigenic stimulation. It is thought to be the site of B memory-cell generation, and contains special dendritic cells which retain antigens on their surface for weeks and perhaps even years.

T T-cell area, or 'paracortex', largely occupied by T cells but through which B cells travel to reach the medulla. It is thought that the dendritic cells here are specialised for presentation of antigen to T cells.

PCV Post-capillary venule; a specialised small venule with high cuboidal endothelium through which lymphocytes leave the blood to enter the paracortex and thence the efferent lymphatic.

SPLEEN

The spleen differs from a lymph node in having no lymphatic drainage, and also in containing large numbers of red cells. In some species it can act as an erythropoietic organ or a reservoir for blood.

TR Trabecula(e); connective tissue structures sheathing the vessels, especially veins.

Spleen continued

T T-cell area; the lymphoid sheath surrounding the arteries is mostly composed of T lymphocytes.

B B-cell area, or lymphoid follicle, typically lying to one side of the lymphoid sheath. Germinal centres are commonly found in the follicle, alongside the follicular artery.

M Marginal zone, the region between the lymphoid areas and the red pulp, where lymphocytes chiefly leave the blood to enter the lymphoid areas, and red cells and plasma cells to enter the red pulp.

RP Red pulp; a reticular meshwork through which blood passes to enter the venous sinusoids, and in which surveillance and removal of damaged red cells is thought to occur. For contrast, the lymphoid areas are sometimes called 'white pulp'. Macrophages in the red pulp and in the marginal zone can retain antigens, as the dendritic cells in the lymph nodes do. As in the medulla of the lymph node, plasma cells are frequent.

S Sinusoids, the large sacs that collect blood for return via the splenic vein.

GUT

The illustration shows a typical Peyer's patch from the ileum, but lymphoid nodules are found up and down the gut, responding to antigens entering through the gut.

PHARYNX

Lymphoid masses, such as tonsils and adenoids, respond to antigens from the nose and throat. Both B and T cells are present and germinal centres are common.

SKIN

Antigens entering via the skin can reach the local lymph node by being taken up in Langerhans cells (**LC** in figure, and see Fig 7), which can pass from the skin to the node, where they probably settle in the T-cell areas.

12 Antibody structure and function

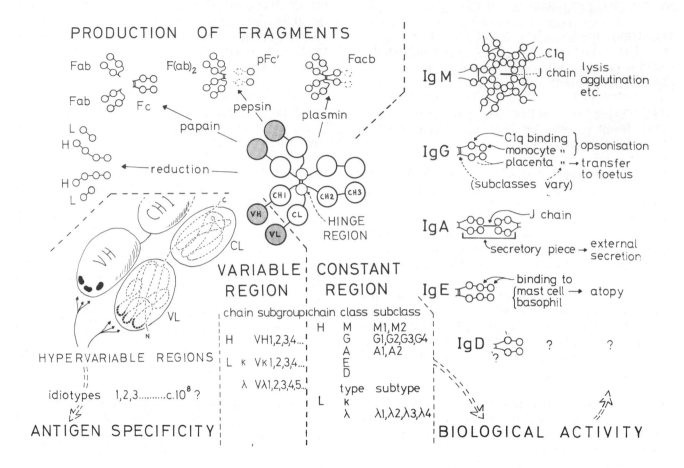

One of the most exciting and intensely studied molecules in existence, **antibody** has yielded most of its secrets to three techniques: separation into fragments by chemical means (top left), amino acid sequencing, and X-ray crystallography. The latter two require the use of completely homogeneous (monoclonal) antibody, which was originally only available in the form of myeloma proteins, the product of malignant B cells, but is nowadays increasingly produced by the hybridoma method.

The basic unit of antibody structure is the homology unit or **domain**, of which a typical molecule (IgG, centre) has twelve, arranged in two heavy and two light (H and L) chains, linked through cysteine residues by disulphide bonds so that the domains lie together in pairs. Variations between the domains of different antibody molecules are responsible for differences in **antigen binding**, which determines **specificity** (lower left) and in **biological activity**, which determines **function** (right). The antigen-binding portion of the

molecule (N-terminal end) shows such heterogeneity that it is known as the **variable** region (shaded). The remainder is relatively **constant**, though with some heterogeneity in the form of **classes** and **subclasses**; the right hand part of the figure shows the different arrangement of the domains in the constant region of the five classes: M, G, A, E and D. The result is a huge variety of molecules able to bring any antigen into contact with any one of several effective disposal mechanisms. The basic molecule (MW about 160,000) can form dimers (IgA, MW 400,000) or pentamers (IgM, MW 900,000; see right-hand side of figure).

There are species differences, especially in the heavy chain subclasses; the examples shown here illustrate human antibodies. Not shown in the figure are the carbohydrate side chains associated with the constant regions, which may constitute up to 12% of the whole molecule but are thought to be involved in secretion rather than function.

Ig Immunoglobulin; a term embracing all globulins with antibody activity, which has replaced 'gammaglobulin' because not all antibodies have gamma electrophoretic mobility.

Fragments produced by chemical treatment:
H,L: Heavy and light chains, which separate under reducing conditions.
Fab: Antigen Binding fragment (papain digestion).
Fc: Crystallisable (because relatively homogeneous) fragment (papain).
F(ab)$_2$: two Fab fragments united by disulphide bonds (pepsin),
pFc': a dimer of CH3 domains (pepsin).
Facb: an Ig molecule lacking CH3 domains (plasmin).

Chains The heavy and two types of light (x, λ) chains are coded for by genes on different chromosomes, but sequence homologies suggest that all Ig domains originated from a common 'precursor' molecule about 110 amino acids long.

Classes Physical, antigenic, and functional variations between constant regions define the five main classes of heavy chain: M, G, A, E and D. These are different molecules all of which are present in all members of most higher species. Brief points of interest are listed below.

IgM is usually the first class of antibody made in a response, and is also thought to have been the first to appear during evolution (see Fig 3). Because its pentameric structure gives it up to ten antigen-combining sites, it is extremely efficient at binding and agglutinating micro-organisms.

IgC, a later development, owes its value to the ability of its Fc portion to bind avidly to Clq (see Fig 5) and to receptors on phagocytic cells (see Fig 8). It also gains access to the extravascular spaces and (via the placenta) to the foetus. In most species, IgG has become further diversified into subclasses (see below).

IgA is the major antibody of secretions such as tears, sweat, and the contents of lungs, gut, urine etc, where, thanks to its secretory piece (see below) it avoids digestion. Its main value is to block the entry of micro-organisms from these external surfaces to the tissues themselves.

IgE is a curious molecule whose main property is to bind to mast cells and promote their degranulation. The good and bad consequences of this are discussed in Fig 27.

IgD appears to function only on the surface of B cells, where it may have some regulatory role.

Subclasses, subtypes, subgroups. Within classes, smaller variations between constant regions define the subclasses found in different molecules of all members of an individual species. The IgG subclasses are generally the most varied. Light chain C region variants of this kind are called 'subtypes' and those in the V regions 'subgroups'. All these variants found in all individuals of a species are called 'isotypic'.

Allotypes By contrast, 'allotypic' variations (not shown in figure) distinguish the Ig molecules of some individuals from some others (c.f. the blood groups). They are genetically determined or perhaps regulated, and mostly occur in the C regions. No biological function has yet been discovered. Unlike blood groups etc, Ig allotypes are expressed singly on individual B cells, a process known as 'allelic exclusion', which shows that only one of the cell's two sets of chromosomes are used for making antibody.

Hypervariable regions Three parts of each of the variable region of heavy and light chains, spaced roughly equally apart in the amino-acid sequence (see figure, lower left) but brought close together as the chain folds, form the antigen-combining site. It is because of the enormous degree of variation in the DNA coding for these regions that the total number of combinations is so high.

Idiotypes In many cases, antibody molecules with different antigen-combining sites can be in turn distinguished by other antibodies made against them. The latter are known as 'anti-idiotypic', implying that each combining site is associated with a different shape, though this is usually not the actual antigen-binding site itself. Anti-idiotypic antibodies are thought to be formed normally and may regulate immune responses (see Fig 15).

Hinge region Both flexibility and proteolytic digestion are facilitated by the repeated proline residues in this part of the molecule. In IgM, the hinge region is as large as a normal domain, and is called CH2, so that the other two constant region domains are called CH3 and CH4; the same may be true for IgE.

J chain A glycopeptide molecule which aids polymerization of IgA and IgM.

Secretory piece A polypeptide produced in epithelial cells and added to IgA dimers to enable them to be transported across the epithelium and secreted into gut, tears, milk etc: where IgA predominates.

Clq The first component of the classical complement sequence, a hexavalent glycoprotein activated by binding to CH2 domains of IgM and some IgG subclasses (in the human, IgG$_1$ and IgG$_3$).

13　Antibody diversification and synthesis

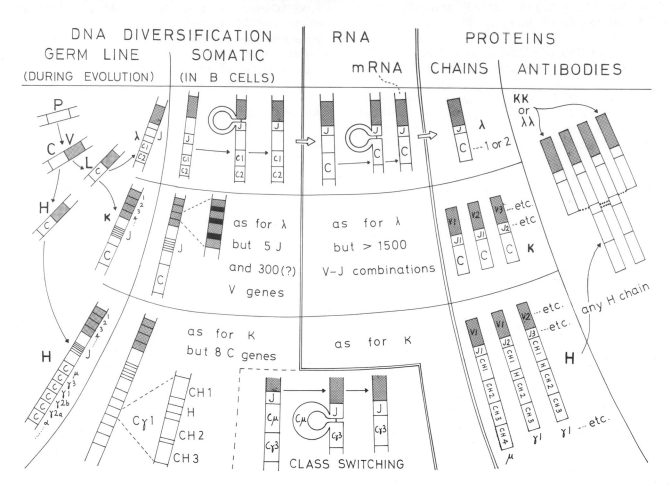

How is the amazing diversity of antibody molecules generated? Much of it arose during evolution; amino acid sequence comparisons suggest that all antibody genes evolved with the vertebrates from a precursor gene coding for a polypeptide about 110 amino acids long (*P*, top left). Repeated gene reduplication, with mutation in the copies, together with occasional translocation to other chromosomes, has led to the present-day **germ-line** gene pool, from which each member of a species inherits an assortment.

Constant region variability (*C* in figure) is mainly restricted to the heavy chain genes (H). But the **variable region** genes (shaded) have generated large numbers of variants, reflected in the 50 or more 'framework' sequences of some light chains (L) such as the K chain in the mouse (centre of figure). Within this large gene pool, the **hypervariable regions** (shown as black bands in the magnified V gene, centre) carry diversification to a unique degree, resulting in a number of different V genes that may exceed 100,000.

Like other proteins, antibodies are synthesised on ribosomes under the direction of messenger RNA, and recent studies using DNA cloning have revealed that further changes occur **somatically** in the B cells, at the level of both DNA and RNA (shown in the figure as loops), mainly involving the excision of unwanted base sequences. Yet more variable region diversification also occurs in the B cells, but it is not yet certain whether this is due to recombination between V genes, to shuffling of a number of small ('mini-') genes, or to mutation.

In the individual B cell, heavy and light chains are synthesised separately (right) and then joined by disulphide bonds before being exported. By a special mechanism, probably also involving excision of DNA, a B cell can retain a particular V gene in combination with a succession of C genes; this is known as class switching' (bottom centre) and is a valuable feature of the antibody response in higher animals.

P Precursor gene; the presumed forerunner of all antibody genes, and of some other proteins involved in cell recognition, such as β2 microglobulin and part of the major histocompatibility antigens.

C,V The constant and variable region precursor genes. Reduplication of the V gene may have started before separation of the heavy and light chain genes.

H,L Heavy and light chain genes. Two translocations presumably led to the present three-chromosome arrangement. Reduplication of the H chain gene subsequently established the basic 3 domain pattern of H chains.

κ, λ Known as kappa and lambda, the two types of L chain gene are on separate chromosomes. The subtypes of λ (C1, C2 in the figure) are reduplications.

Classes, subclasses In the H chain gene, further reduplications of the C gene led to the five classes (M, G, A, E, and D) found in most species. Subsequent reduplication of G seems to have occurred since speciation; i.e. mouse G subclasses are quite different from human. The order of some of the mouse C genes is now fairly certain (see figure, bottom left).

J The J, or 'joining' region, whose gene is brought by successive excisions, into contact with both V and C genes. The process is shown in the figure (top) for the mouse λ gene, which is unusual in having little or no V gene diversity. In the embryo about 3000 bases separate the V and J genes, and this intervening sequence, or 'intron', is excised in the DNA of the B cell. However the other intron, about 1000 bases long, between the J and C genes is removed in a completely different way: by excision and 'splicing' of the messenger RNA. Thus the gene itself is never a continuous whole, but 'split', a surprising feature of many other genes too. For κ and H chains, the process is more complicated, because of the existence of numerous V genes and more than one J gene (5 for the mouse κ chain). Probably any V gene can combine with any J, and the J region makes some contribution to combining-site diversity, particularly in H chains.

Hypervariable regions The most interesting and controversial process of all is that by which the full range of antigen-combining sites is generated. Again considering the mouse κ chain, there appear to be 300 – 350 V genes, arranged in about 50 groups. However the amino-acid variability in the hypervariable regions suggests a much higher total number of possible sequences. Three somatic events have been postulated to explain this. (1) Recombination between different V genes, with exchange of DNA sequences; perhaps the existence of the groups facilitates this; (2) The three hypervariable regions and the four framework regions on either side could each be coded by separate genes (the minigene theory); clearly this would allow an enormous scope for new combinations. (3) Occasional point mutations could also introduce variability; at one time this was in fact thought to be the source of all somatic diversification.

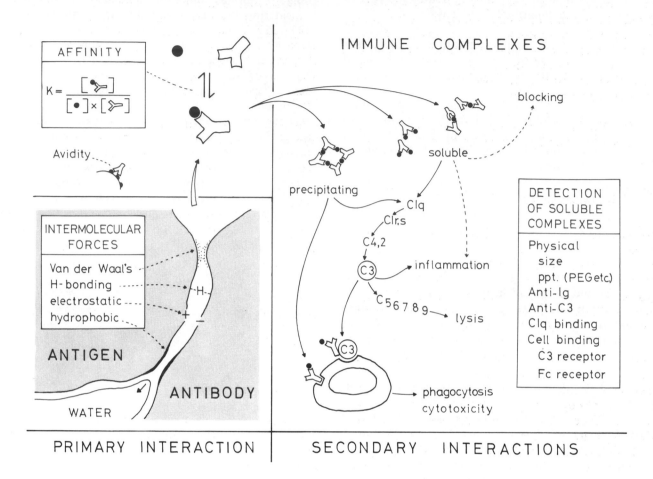

The primary function of antibody is to combine with antigen (left), which alone may be enough to neutralise, for example, toxins or some viruses. But a secondary interaction of the antibody molecule with another effector agent (e.g. complement, phagocytic cells: right) is usually required to dispose of larger antigens such as bacteria. The importance of these secondary interactions is shown by the fact that deficiency of complement or myeloid cells can be almost as serious as deficiency of antibody itself (see Fig 33).

The ability of a particular antibody to combine with one antigen rather than another is referred to as its 'specificity', and resides in the part of the Fab portion known as the **'combining site'**, a cleft formed largely by the hypervariable regions of heavy and light chains (see Fig 12). The closer the fit between this site and a given small piece (or **'determinant'**) of the antigen, the stronger will be the non-covalent forces (hydrophobic,

electrostatic, etc: lower left) between them, and the higher the **'affinity'** (top left). When both combining sites can interact with the same antigen (e.g. a cell), the bond has a greatly increased strength, which in this case is referred to as 'avidity'.

The combination of antigen and antibody is called an **'immune complex'**; this may be small (soluble) or large (precipitating), depending on the nature and proportions of antigen and antibody (top right). The usual fate of complexes is to be removed by phagocytic cells, through the interaction of the Fc portion of the antibody with complement and with cell-surface receptors (bottom centre and Fig 8). However in some cases complexes may persist in circulation and cause inflammatory damage to organs (see Fig 28) or inhibit useful immunity, e.g. to tumours or parasites. The detection of complexes and the identification of the antigen in them is therefore important and numerous techniques are available.

ANTIGEN-ANTIBODY INTERACTION

The combining site of antibody is a cleft roughly 3 x 1 x 1 nm (the size of 5 or 6 sugar units), though there is evidence that antigens may bind to larger, or even separate, parts of the variable region. Binding depends on a close 3-dimensional fit, allowing weak intermolecular forces to overcome the normal repulsion between molecules.

Van der Waal's forces attract all molecules through their electron clouds, but only act at extremely close range.

Hydrogen bonding, e.g. between $-NH_2$ and $-OH$ groups, is another weak force.

Electrostatic attraction between antibody and antigen molecules with a net opposite charge is sometimes quite strong.

Hydrophobic regions on antigen and antibody will tend to be attracted in an aqueous environment; this is probably the strongest force between them.

Affinity is normally expressed as the association constant under equilibrium conditions. A value of 10^3 litres/mole would be considered low, while high affinity antibody can reach 10^{10} 1/m and over — several orders of magnitude higher than most enzyme-substrate interactions. In practice, it is often **avidity** which is measured, and even with monovalent antigens a serum can only be assigned an average affinity. Average affinity tends to increase with time after antigenic stimulation, probably thorough cell selection. High affinity antibodies are more effective in most cases, but low affinity antibodies persist too, and may have certain advantages (re-usability, resistance to tolerance?)

IMMUNE COMPLEXES

Under conditions of antigen or antibody excess, small ('soluble') complexes tend to predominate, but with roughly equivalent amounts of antigen and antibody, precipitates form, probably by lattice formation. In the presence of complement (i.e. in fresh serum) only small complexes are formed; in fact C3 can actually solubilise larger complexes.

Blocking of T-cell or antibody-mediated killing by complexes in (respectively) antigen or antibody excess, may account for some of the unresponsiveness to tumours or parasite infections.

C1q the first component of complement, binds to the Fc portion of complexed antibody, possibly under the influence of a conformational change in the shape of the Ig molecule, although some workers hold that occupation of both combining sites (i.e. of IgG) is all that is needed. Activation of the 'classical' complement pathway follows.

Inflammation Breakdown products of C3 and C5, through interaction with mast cells, polymorphs, etc, are responsible for the vascular damage which is a feature of 'immune complex diseases'.

Lysis e.g. of bacteria, requires the complete complement sequence. Sometimes the C567 unit moves away from the original site of antibody binding, activates C8 and 9, and causes lysis of innocent cells, (e.g. red cells); this is known as 'reactive lysis'.

Phagocytosis by macrophages, polymorphs, eosinophils, etc, is the normal fate of large complexes. In general, the antibody classes and subclasses which bind to Fc receptors also bind to complement, making them strongly opsonic, but the Fc and C3 receptors are quite distinct; IgM, for example, binds to complement much more than to cells.

Cytotoxicity When antibody bound to a cell or micro-organism makes contact with Fc receptors, the result may be killing rather than phagocytosis. Cells able to do this include macrophages, monocytes, and the lymphocyte-like 'K' cell (see Fig 9). The importance of this type of 'antibody-mediated cytotoxicity' *in vivo* is controversial.

Detection of soluble complexes
Complexes tend to be of large size (e.g. in the ultracentrifuge or gradients), and to precipitate in the cold ('cryoprecipitation') and in polyethylene glycol (PEG). Since they contain Ig, complexes react with anti-Ig antibodies (e.g. rheumatoid factor). Their reaction with C1q is used in a number of sensitive assays, and the presence of C3 can be deduced from reaction with anti-C3 antibody (immunoconglutinin) and binding to cells with C3 receptors, such as the Raji cell line. In general, these assays agree, but some complexes do not fix complement yet are precipitated by PEG, while some tests can be complicated by the presence of other large molecules. Therefore several tests may need to be done in parallel.

15 The antibody response

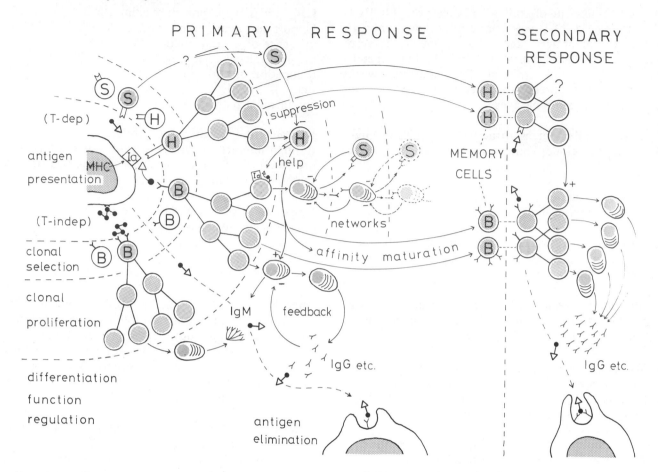

One of the most dramatic manifestations of adaptive immunity is the **antibody response**, in which a small pre-existing B cell population (centre left, shaded) already committed to a particular antigen by the possession of complementary surface Ig, is stimulated to divide and secrete large amounts of specific antibody, usually leading to the elimination of the stimulating antigen and leaving the body 'primed' for an even more effective response upon subsequent contact (right).

Antigens can be thought of as **'haptenic'** groups (black circles) which interact with antibody-combining sites, and **'carrier'** determinants (triangles) which enable them to trigger B cells into a response. Generally this is because they stimulate specific **T helper cells** (H, shaded), but some large polymeric molecules are carriers in the absence of T cells; these constitute 'T-independent' antigens (lower left). Once triggered, B cells are subject to a variety of regulatory influences (centre) involving both specific and non-specific (not shown here) factors, anti-idiotype responses, etc, whose relative importance is not yet clear. Most of the cell interactions depicted here occur in the spleen and lymph nodes, but antibody can also be formed locally in many other sites.

It should be emphasised that even small, well-defined antigenic determinants usually stimulate a heterogeneous population of B cells, each producing antibody of slightly different specificity and affinity. In the **secondary response**, average affinity tends to be higher (probably by cell selection), precursor cells more numerous, and Ig class more varied — which together make secondary responses very much more effective.

Macrophages play such a central role, both in triggering T and B cells and in eliminating the antigen, that the antibody response can almost be regarded as a roundabout means of improving macrophage function. However there is a suggestion that the cells which present antigen may not be the same as the ones that phagocytose it; probably macrophages will turn out, like lymphocytes, to be made up of interesting subpopulations (see Fig 7).

Antigen presentation Most, perhaps all, antigens require presentation before they can trigger lymphocytes. This is performed by special cells in spleen, lymph nodes, skin etc (see Fig 7) and usually involves an association between antigen and certain products of the Major Histocompatibility Complex (**MHC**), called the I antigens (**Ia** in figure, and see Fig 17 for more details).

Haptens (black circles in the figure) are chemical groupings against which antibody can be made, but only if they are coupled to a carrier (see below). Typical haptens are substituted phenol rings, small peptides, sugars etc.

Carriers (white triangles in the figure) are typically large proteins but cells, micro-organisms etc can function in the same way, which is to enlist 'help'. Note that it is perfectly possible for the same portion (or 'determinant') of the antigen to function as both a carrier and a hapten, though not to provide help for itself.

T-dep T-dependent antigens include the vast majority of proteins, cells etc, which cannot induce antibody unless helper T cells are present.

T-indep T-independent antigens are large molecules with repeating identical determinants, mainly polysaccharides. They do not need T cells to induce antibody, but most still require macrophages.

B B lymphocytes, which recognise antigenic determinants through their surface Ig receptor: each B cell bears receptors, and synthesises Ig, of a single specificity. The B cells that respond to T-dependent and T-independent antigens are probably different subpopulations ('B1, B2').

H Helper T cell, whose recognition of carrier determinants in association with Ia on first the antigen-presenting cell and subsequently the B lymphocyte, provides 'help' (see below) and permits antibody responses to T-dependent antigens. It is not clear whether this recognition involves one or two separate receptors, nor exactly what the structure of the receptor is (this goes for all other types of T cell too).

S Suppressor T cell, also responding to carrier determinants but acting to diminish the effect of helper T cells.

Clonal selection; clonal proliferation Interaction of antigen and surface Ig causes division of the appropriate B cell, forming a 'clone' of identical cells. The same probably occurs with helper T cells (and perhaps with suppressors?). Because of the non-specific factors also involved, cell division is not strictly limited to specific B and T cells. A few antigens are in fact strong non-specific stimulators of cell division, or 'mitogens'.

Help Partly by cell contact and partly through the release of 'helper factors', helper T cells stimulate the production of antibody by B cells. Though not fully characterised, these factors include both non-antigen-specific and antigen-specific molecules, the latter apparently carrying both MHC products (I antigens, see Fig 17) and immunoglobulin V regions; they may or may not be identical to the T cell receptor. Helper cells play little part in B cell proliferation, but may assist in Ig class switching and the maturation of affinity. Some antigens e.g. lipopolysaccharides, can substitute for T-cell effects.

Suppression can also be either specific or non-specific, and can act at the level of both the helper T cell and the B cell itself. Suppressor factors appear to resemble helper factors, except that a different MHC product may be involved. However the nature of all these factors is still highly controversial.

IgM Most T-independent, and the earliest T-dependent, antibody is IgM.

IgG IgG, IgA, and IgE are relatively more dependent on T-cell help than IgM. It is thought that most B cells start by making IgM and then switch to another class.

Feedback Once IgG is made, it tends to inhibit further IgM, IgE, etc, but the mechanism is still obscure and may involve T cells and/or macrophages.

Networks It has been hypothesised, and subsequently shown, that antibody idiotypes (i.e. the unique features related to specificity) can themselves act as antigens, and promote both B and T cell responses against the cells carrying them, so that the immune response progressively damps itself out. This leads to the fascinating concept of a network of anti-idiotype receptors corresponding to all the antigens an animal can respond to—a sort of 'internal image' of its external environment. However the actual role of networks in regulating ordinary antibody responses is not yet clear, nor is that of suppressor T cells. In practice the single most important element in regulating antibody production is probably the removal of the antigen itself.

Affinity The average bond strength between antibody and the inducing antigen increases during the response; probably this is due to progressive selection of the 'best-fitting' B cells, but molecular mechanisms have also been proposed.

Memory cells Instead of differentiating into antibody-producing plasma cells, some B cells persist as memory cells, whose increased number and rapid response underlies the highly augmented secondary response. Memory B cells differ slightly from their precursors (in surface Ig, adherence, recirculation, etc). The generation of memory cells appears to take place in germinal centres, and to be somehow linked to T cells, since T-independent responses do not show memory. However T-dependent memory cells can be generated in the absence of T cells, so it may be the B cells themselves which are different (see B1, B2, above).

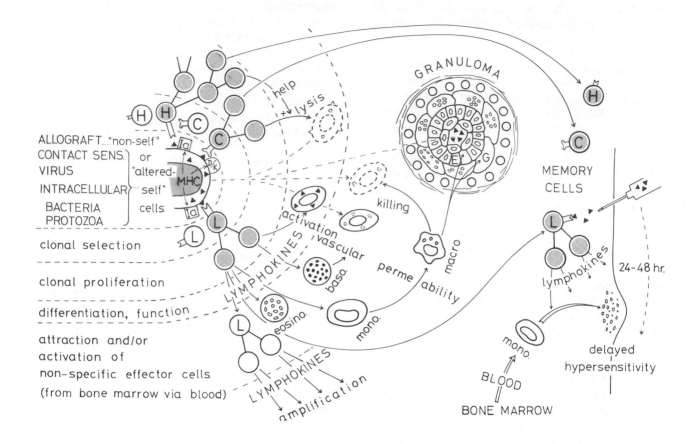

As regards adaptive immune responses not involving antibody, terminology is confusing. The usual term **'cell-mediated'** (i.e. not humoral) is not strictly accurate, since some non-antibody mediators ('lymphokines') do in fact circulate. **'Delayed hypersensitivity'**, which is often used synonymously, merely describes the slow appearance of secondary responses in the skin (right), and dates from the time when antibody responses were detected by 'immediate hypersensitivity'; subtle differences in time course of delayed responses (tuberculin type, Jones-Mote type, etc) probably in fact reflect quite different sets of cells and mediators.

The common links between the responses shown in the figure are the requirement of **T cells** and the presentation of antigen (black triangles) in the form of living cells — either foreign (e.g. grafted), or containing live micro-organisms, or chemically modified — and therefore in association with other cell-surface antigens. Once again, it is the products of

the **MHC** which are involved here (emphasising the absolutely central role of this genetic complex in all T cell responses). Foreign or virus-infected cells may be directly lysed and killed by cytotoxic T cells (**C**; top left), whilst larger micro-organisms that survive within macrophages stimulate a different kind of T cell (**L**; centre left) which acts to increase the efficiency of macrophages and other non-lymphoid cells (centre). The interesting way in which different MHC antigens are recognised by different types of T cell is discussed in more detail in Fig 17.

Not shown in the figure are the various suppressor cells which are thought to modulate these T cell functions, rather as they do the antibody response; they may partly explain the frequently inverse relationship of antibody and cell-mediated responses, though this may also be due to direct blocking — e.g. of cell-mediated responses by antigen-antibody complexes.

Allograft A graft of tissue from a genetically different member of the same species; e.g. a human kidney (see Fig 31 for details).

Contact sens Substances (e.g. DNCB, poison ivy) that bind to skin and other cells can give rise to contact sensitivity.

Virus; intracellular bacteria, protozoa Cells that harbour micro-organisms usually display altered surface antigens so that, as in the two above examples, the cell has both 'self' and 'non-self' features, to which T cells are particularly responsive.

H Helper T cell, responding to 'altered-self' determinants and helping cytotoxic T cells. Most of the proliferation when allogeneic lymphocytes are mixed ('mixed lymphocyte reaction') is due to these cells. Like the antibody-helper T cells (see Fig 15), they recognise antigen in association with **Ia** products of the MHC; indeed these two types of cell may be essentially the same.

C Cytotoxic T cells, which recognise major histocompatibility antigens, or antigens (e.g. viruses) associated with them, and induce irreversible lytic changes in the target cell. They differ from helper T cells both in their surface antigens (e.g. LyT, see Fig 9) and in the MHC products they recognise: in the case of the mouse (illustrated here) the **D** and **K** antigens, equivalent to the human A, B and C (see Fig 31).

L Lymphokine-producing cell; probably a group of T cell subpopulations that respond to antigen by releasing mediators that attract or activate other cells. Sometimes referred to as 'delayed hypersensitivity T cells', they have many features in common with helper T cells (same LyT antigens, same MHC product recognised).

Clonal selection, proliferation All the above T cells respond by expansion of specific precursors into a clone, but the precise nature of their specific receptors is not known.

Lymphokines A large group of non-antigen specific factors produced by T (and sometimes B) cells, with different biological effects, concerned essentially with mediating interactions between cells. Some of the best known act on macrophages, but there are also interactions in the opposite direction — i.e. by macrophages on lymphocytes and the present tendency is to refer to all such 'interaction' molecules as **interleukins** (IL, see below). In general these factors are presumed to act only at high concentration, and thus to help localise cell-mediated immune responses to the vicinity of the antigen. Examples of this type of factor are:

1. Made by lymphocytes
   Macrophage migration inhibitory factor (MIF)
   Macrophage activating factor (MAF)
   Eosinophil chemotactic and activating factors
   Mitogenic factor (MF)
   T cell growth factor (TCGF = IL2)
   Interferon (type 2 or 'immune')
   Lymphotoxin (LT) ⎤
   Proliferation inhibitory factor (PIF) ⎦ — may be identical?

2. Made by macrophages (sometimes called 'monokines')
   Lymphocyte activating factor (LAF = IL 1)
   Interferon (type 1)
   Cytoxin

Activation Some macrophages cannot kill intracellular organisms (e.g. L. monocytogenes, T. gondii) unless activated by T cell products.

Baso Basophil activation by T cells may in turn lead to increased vascular permeability and further cell migration into the tissues.

Eosino Eosinophil production and migration appear to be partly under T cell control.

Mono, Macro The blood monocytes are the principal source of macrophages in cell-mediated lesions, being attracted there and activated by lymphokines.

E Epithelioid cell; a macrophage specialised for enzyme secretion.

G Giant cell, produced by fusion of several macrophages.

Granuloma Undegradeable material (e.g. tubercle bacilli, streptococcal cell walls, talc) may be sequestered in a focus of concentric macrophages also containing some lymphocytes and eosinophils.

17 Genetic control of immunity

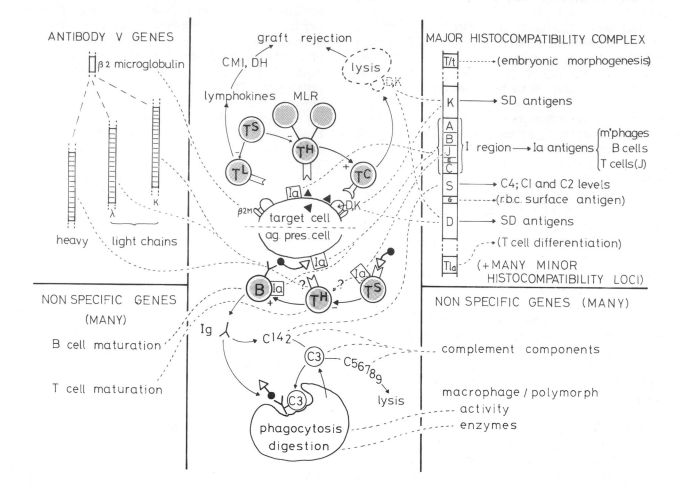

To depict the genetic control of immunity in simple terms would be misleading! Numerous genes (left and right panels in figure) affect immune performance (centre panel: antibody response, lower half; cell-mediated responses, upper half), expressing themselves (broken lines) through all components of the immune system.

The most important in relation to general susceptibility to infection are the genes directing the production and maturation of lymphocytes and phagocytic cells (bottom left, bottom right). Some genetic complement defects also predispose to infection. Idiotypic differences in the repertoire of immunoglobulin variable genes (top left) can influence antibody specificity, but these usually show up only with very well defined antigens.

Most fascinating of all are the wide range of cell-surface structures coded by highly polymorphic genes in the **Major Histocompatibility Complex** (top right), which were first detected through their effect on

transplant rejection (see Fig 31), but which play a decisive part in all responses involving T cells, since most T cells appear to be programmed to recognise **'altered-self-MHC'** products. The example shown is from the mouse, but the MHC in all mammalian species appears broadly similar, though there may be differences in the placing of the I region. It is suspected that this whole complex evolved by reduplication of a primitive 'receptor' gene rather as the immunoglobulin genes did.

The human MHC, known as HLA ('human leucocyte antigen') because its gene products were originally identified on white blood cells, is currently attracting great interest on account of the strong association between individual HLA antigens and diseases. This may reflect the ability and inability of T cells to respond to particular HLA antigen-virus combinations, or to actual resemblances between HLA and micro-organisms, leading to 'tolerance' (see Fig 18); there are also other more complicated theories.

Antibody V genes   The variable regions of the heavy and two light chain genes contain all the information available for the construction of antibody combining sites.

β2 Microglobulin   A small serum protein (MW 11800) also present on cell surfaces in association with MHC components (see below). It probably has a common genetic ancestry with immunoglobulins.

Major Histocompatibility Complex (MHC)   A genetic region found in all higher animals, whose products control graft rejection ('histocompatibility') and most other immune responses. In the human it is called HLA, in the mouse (shown in figure) H2. H2 is formed of three major subregions: D and K, whose gene products are expressed on most cells and detectable by alloantibodies ('serologically defined'; SD) and I, whose products, known as Ia antigens, were originally detectable only by cell-mediated tests ('lymphocyte defined'; LD). In the human, A, B, and C antigens correspond to D and K, and D to mouse I. To avoid this sort of confusion, the present trend is to call all SD antigens Class I and all LD antigens Class II, regardless of species. It is interesting that between and on either side of these regions are other genes also affecting cell differentiation or recognition, and, oddly enough, some of the genes for complement components.

I region   This large central stretch of the mouse MHC can be subdivided by breeding experiments into subregions (A, B, J, E, C). There is a suggestion that the A region is involved in help and the J region in suppression.

MHC gene products. D and **K** antigens are glycoproteins with a two-chain structure rather like Ig; β2 microglobulin plays the part of 'light chain', and the heavy chains (MW 45,000 also show some sequence homology with Ig. **Ia** antigens are less well worked out, but appear to have two subunits, of MW about 36,000 and 26,000.

Minor histocompatibility loci   In the mouse, many other genes also control graft rejection. Named H1, H3, 4, 5 . . . they are simpler, and their influence weaker, than H2, to which they stand in a relationship like that of the minor blood group antigens to ABO. A gene on the Y chromosome affects the survival of male grafts in female recipients in the mouse, and probably also in the human.

B   B lymphocyte, carrying both specific immunoglobulin (Ig) and Ia antigens coded for by the I region of the MHC.

T^H   Helper T cell, recognising antigen via a receptor of uncertain nature, possibly composed of both MHC-coded products and Ig heavy chains. T cells appear to 'see' antigens in conjunction with Ia antigen on macrophages and B cells, so that what they recognise is influenced by the precise nature of the Ia antigens and thus of the animal's own genetic make-up.

T^S   Suppressor T cell, acting either via the helper T cell or directly on the B cell to specifically inhibit antibody production. It is not known exactly what suppressor T cells recognise, but it involves determinants coded for by the J region of the MHC.

T^C   Cytotoxic T cell, able to lyse foreign cells, virus-infected cells, etc. Cytotoxic T cells apparently 'see' virus antigens etc: in conjunction with products of the D and K regions of the MHC.

T^L   Lymphokine-secreting T cell, the presumptive initiator of delayed hypersensitivity and other cell-mediated responses. Since these responses also involve Ia antigens on the presenting cell, either the T^L cell, or perhaps its helper cell, probably recognises antigen in conjunction with Ia, as the antibody-helper T cell does.

MLR   Mixed lymphocyte reaction, a proliferative response to MHC products, predominately Ia, convenient for detecting LD antigen differences.

HLA-ASSOCIATED DISEASES

Far the most striking is the group of arthropathies involving the sacro-iliac joint (Ankylosing Spondylitis, Reiter's Disease etc) where one HLA antigen (B 27) is found in up to 95% of cases — nearly 20 times its frequency in the general population. But numerous other diseases, including almost all the autoimmune diseases, show a statistically significant association with particular HLA antigens, or groups of antigens. The tendency of HLA antigens (for example A1 and B8) to 'stay together' instead of segregating normally is called 'linkage disequilibrium' and may imply that such combinations are of survival value, perhaps because they increase resistance to diseases or, alternatively, because they reduce the risk of hypersensitivity. This whole field is in an exciting stage of evolution.

18 Tolerance

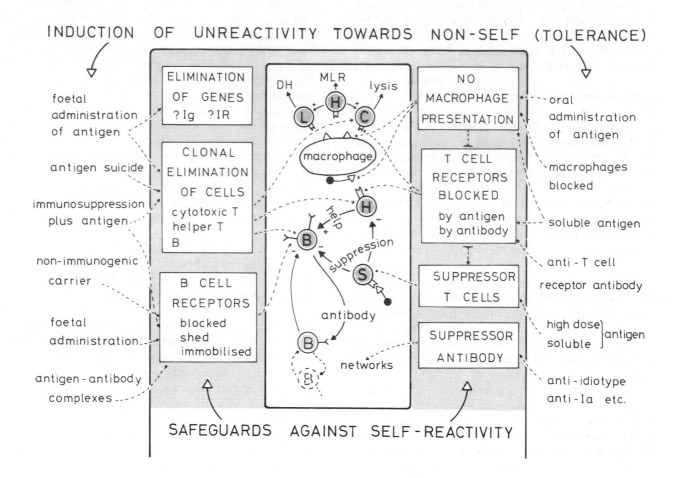

The evolution of recognition systems that initiate destruction of 'non-self' material obviously carries with it the need for safeguards to prevent damage to 'self'. This is largely a **lymphocyte** problem, since most non-lymphoid defence mechanisms (phagocytosis, direct activation of C3, lysozyme, interferon) are normally active against components exclusive to micro-organisms, or against already damaged 'self' material.

Within the lymphoid system, immune responses are protected against self-reactivity at many levels. In the figure, the centre panel depicts cell-mediated (top) and antibody (bottom) mechanisms, and the shaded panels on either side show the principal safeguards. It used to be assumed that elimination of potentially self-reactive clones (centre, left) was the basis of all unresponsiveness to self, but other more complex regulatory mechanisms are now also recognised. Failure of these mechanisms can lead to self-damaging immune responses (see Autoimmunity; Fig 30).

In certain circumstances (extreme left and right), these safeguarding mechanisms can also be triggered by normally antigenic 'non-self' materials, in which case these are subsequently treated essentially like 'self', a state known as **tolerance**, which may on occasions be useful (e.g. organ transplantation). Note that tolerance is by definition antigen-specific, and distinct from the non-specific unresponsiveness induced by damage to the immune system as a whole (see Immunosuppression; Fig 32). Note also that some immunologists prefer to restrict the term 'tolerance' to proved cases of clonal elimination; unfortunately clonal elimination is usually rather difficult to prove.

SAFEGUARDS AGAINST SELF REACTIVITY

Elimination of genes   It has been suggested that self-reactive cells are continually stimulated by self-antigen until, by mutation of receptor genes, they lose self-reactivity. (No evidence).

Clonal elimination   A cornerstone of Burnet's Clonal Selection Theory, following from the prediction (since confirmed) that individual lymphocytes were restricted in their antigen recognition. Some self-reactive cells may be eliminated in the thymus (T) and the bone marrow (B), but evidence has been difficult to obtain.

Macrophage presentation is essential for most immune responses. Macrophages may recognise 'self' cell surface antigens and fail to present them to lymphocytes.

B cell receptors (immunoglobulin) may be occupied by antigen in a non-triggering form. Foetal B cells may shed their Ig and fail to replace it — effectively a form of clonal elimination. Note, however, that B cells able to bind some self antigens (e.g. thyroglobulin) are found in normal animals.

T cell receptors often appear to lose their triggering function in the presence of the specific antigen in soluble form. When cultured in the absence of 'self' serum, cytotoxic T cells can sometimes develop into 'self-killers', suggesting a serum blocking factor.

Suppressor T cells have been postulated to recognise and inhibit self-reactive lymphocytes, but the evidence is controversial.

Suppressor antibody against Ig idiotypes might help to inhibit self-reactive B cells that have escaped other controls. Antibody against cell surfaces might, if not itself destructive, protect against other forms of attack.

INDUCTION OF UNREACTIVITY TOWARDS NON-SELF

Soluble antigen is generally more tolerogenic than aggregated or particulate, mainly because macrophages do not 'present' it, but perhaps in addition becasue it can block lymphocyte receptors and stimulate suppressor T cells.

High doses of antigen are usually more tolerogenic, though repeated low doses can also induce tolerance, but only in T cells. As a rule, T cell tolerance is easier to induce and lasts longer than B cell tolerance.

Oral administration   Antigens absorbed through the gut are first 'seen' by liver macrophages, which remove immunogenic aggregates etc, leaving soluble 'tolerogen'. Some cases may also be due to high levels of IgA, which are said to inhibit other Ig classes.

Foetal (or neonatal) administration probably operates by a combination of clonal elimination and deficient macrophage presentation, but foetal B cells may also be particularly tolerizable because of differences in the way their Ig receptors are replaced (see above).

Non-immunogenic carriers, such as 'self' material or non-degradeable molecules (e.g. D-amino acid polypeptides), can confer tolerogenicity on haptens that, on normal carriers, are antigenic. This idea has been tried in allergy, to switch off specific IgE responses.

Antigen suicide   Antigens coupled to toxic drugs, radioisotopes etc, may home onto specific T or B cells and kill them without exposing other cells to danger. A field with an exciting future.

Antibody   Tolerance induced by antibody is sometimes called 'enhancement', from its ability to increase the growth of grafts, tumours, etc. In theory, antibody against T or B cell receptors ('anti-idiotype') or against the structures they recognise (e.g. anti-Ia) can interfere with the induction of the normal immune response.

19 Anti-microbial immunity: a general scheme

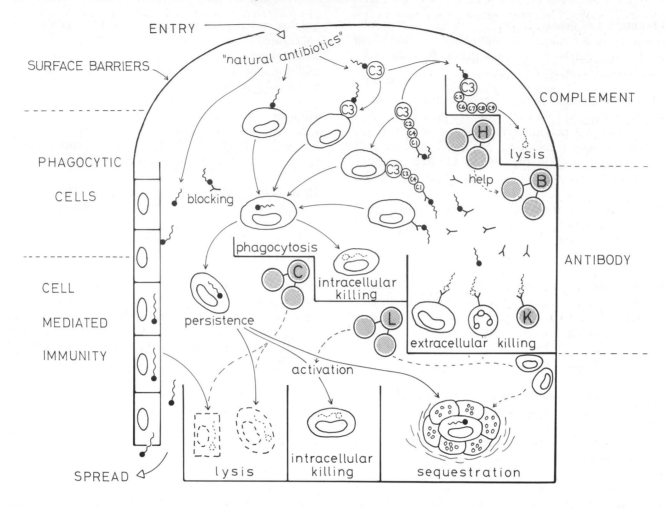

In responding to microbial infection, the immune system can unfortunately only detect *foreignness*, and not *pathogenicity*. Would-be parasitic micro-organisms that penetrate the barriers of skin or mucous membranes (top) have to run the gauntlet of four main recognition systems: **complement** (top right), **phagocytic cells** (centre), **antibody** (right), and **cell-mediated immunity** (bottom), and their often interacting effector mechanisms. Unless primed by previous contact with the appropriate antigen, antibody and cell-mediated responses do not come into action for several days, whereas complement and phagocytic cells, being ever-present, act within minutes. There are also (top centre) specialised **natural** elements, such as lysozyme, interferon etc, which act more or less non-specifically, much as **antibiotics** do.

Generally speaking, complement and antibody are most active against micro-organisms free in the blood or tissues, whilst cell-mediated responses are most active against those that seek refuge in cells (left). But which mechanism, if any, is actually effective depends largely on the tactics of the micro-organism itself. Successful parasites are those able to evade, resist, or inhibit the relevant immune mechanisms, as illustrated in the five following figures.

Entry Many micro-organisms enter the body through wounds or bites, but others live on the skin or mucous membranes of the intestine, respiratory tract etc, and are thus technically outside the body.

Surface barriers Skin and mucous membranes are to some extent protected by acid pH, enzymes, mucus, and other antimicrobial secretions.

Natural antibiotics Produced largely by macrophages, the antibacterial enzyme **lysozyme** (see Fig 20) and the antiviral **interferons** (see Fig 21), are responsible for a good deal of the natural immunity to what would otherwise be pathogenic organisms, and it is likely that other similar agents remain to be discovered. However this type of protection is obviously restricted by the need to avoid damage to self material.

C3 Complement is activated directly ('alternative pathway') by many micro-organisms, leading to their lysis or phagocytosis. The same effect can also be achieved when C3 is activated by antibody ('classical pathway'; see Fig 5).

H Helper T cell, responding to 'carrier' determinants and stimulating antibody synthesis by B cells. Viruses, bacteria, protozoa, and worms have all been shown to function as fairly strong carriers.

B Antibody formation by B lymphocytes is an almost universal feature of infection, of great diagnostic as well as protective value.

Blocking Where micro-organisms need to enter cells, antibody may block this by combining with their specific attachment site. Malaria and most viruses are examples. IgA in the intestine acts mainly in this way.

Phagocytosis by polymorphonuclear leucocytes or macrophages is the ultimate fate of most unsuccessful organisms. Both C3 and antibody tremendously improve this by attaching the microbe to the phagocytic cell through C3 or Fc receptors on the latter; this is known as 'opsonisation'.

Intracellular killing Once inside the phagocytic cell, most organisms are killed and degraded by lysosomal enzymes. In certain cases, 'activation' of macrophages by T cells may be needed to trigger the killing process.

Extracellular killing Monocytes, polymorphs, and 'K' cells can kill antibody-coated cells *in vitro*, without phagocytosis; however it is not clear how much this actually happens *in vivo*.

K 'Killer' cell: a lymphocyte-like (but not proved to be lymphoid) cell able to kill tumour cells extracellularly *in vitro*, through attachment of specific antibody to its receptors for the Fc region of IgG.

Persistence Several important viruses, bacteria, and protozoa can survive inside macrophages, where they resist killing. Other organisms survive within cells of muscle, liver, brain etc. In such cases antibody cannot attack them and cell-mediated responses are the only hope.

C Cytotoxic T cell, specialised for killing, by lysis, 'self' cells altered by viruses etc, and also allogeneic (e.g. grafted) cells.

L Lymphokine-producing T cell, important in attracting and activating monocytes, eosinophils etc, and in 'delayed hypersensitivity'.

Sequestration Micro-organisms which cannot be killed (e.g. some mycobacteria) or products which cannot be degraded (e.g. streptococcal cell walls) can be walled off by the formation of a granuloma by macrophages, often aided by cell-mediated immune responses.

Spread Successful micro-organisms must be able to leave the body and infect another one. Coughs and sneezes, faeces, and insect bites are the commonest modes of spread.

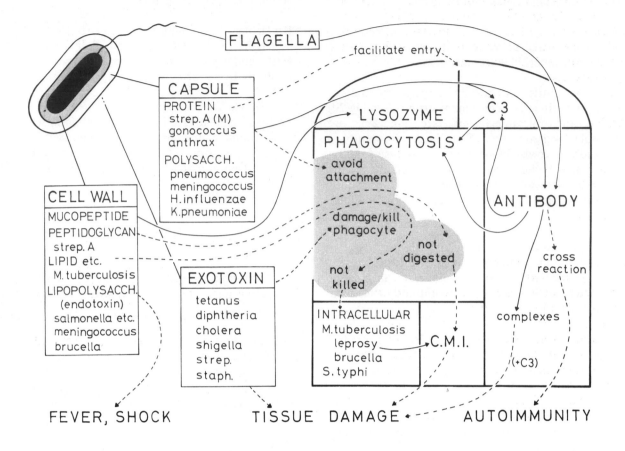

The usual destiny of unsuccessful bacteria is death by **phagocytosis** (centre; shaded); survival therefore entails avoidance of this fate. The main ways in which a bacterium (top left) can achieve this lie in the **capsule** (affecting attachment), the **cell wall** (affecting digestion), and the release of **exotoxins** (which damage phagocytic and other cells). Fortunately most capsules and toxins are strongly antigenic and antibody overcomes many of their effects; this is the basis of the majority of antibacterial vaccines. In the figure, processes beneficial to the bacteria or harmful to the host are shown in broken lines.

On the host side, the 'natural antibiotic' **lysozyme** represents perhaps the farthest point achieved in elaborating substances that attack bacteria but not host cells (until the antibiotic era; it is interesting that both lysozyme and penicillin were discovered by Fleming).

In the long run, no parasite that seriously damages or kills its host can count on its own survival, so that adaptation, which can be quite rapid in bacteria, tends to be in the direction of decreased virulence. But infections that are well adapted to their normal host can occasionally be highly virulent to man; plague (rats) and brucellosis (cattle) are examples of this ('zoonosis').

CELL WALL

All bacteria have strong cell walls, basically composed of **mucopeptides** containing muramic acid, susceptible to lysozyme. In addition different species, mainly Gram-negative, have special **lipids, lipopolysaccharides**, or mucopolysaccharides (e.g. **peptidoglycan**) which confer resistance to lysozyme and phagocytosis.

FLAGELLA

the main agents of bacterial motility, contain highly antigenic proteins (the 'H antigens' of typhoid etc) giving rise to immobilising antibody.

CAPSULE

Many bacteria owe their virulence to capsules, which protect them from contact with phagocytes. Most are large branched polysaccharide molecules, but some are protein. It is interesting that many of these capsular polysaccharides, and also some proteins from flagella, are T-independent antigens (see Fig 15). Since T-independent antibody is thought to have preceded the T-dependent type in evolution (see Fig 3), this fits in with the idea that bacteria were the main driving force for the development of the antibody-forming system.

EXOTOXIN

(as distinct from the **endotoxin** of cell walls). Gram-positive bacteria often secrete proteins with destructive effects on phagocytes, local tissues, the CNS etc; frequently these are the cause of death.

BACTERIA

In the figure, bacteria are given their popular rather than their proper taxonomic names. Some individual aspects of interest are listed below:

Strep Streptococcus, classified either by haemolytic exotoxins (α, β, λ) or cell wall antigens (groups A-Q). Group A, β-haemolytic are the most pathogenic, possessing capsules (M protein) that attach to mucous membranes but resist phagocytosis, numerous exotoxins (whence scarlet fever), indigestible cell walls causing severe cell-mediated reactions, antigens that cross-react with cardiac muscle (rheumatic fever), and a tendency to nephritogenic immune complexes.

Staph Staphylococcus. Antiphagocytic factors include the fibrin-forming enzyme coagulase and protein A, which binds to the Fc portion of IgG, blocking opsonisation. Numerous other toxins make staphylocci highly destructive, abscess-forming organisms.

Pneumococcus, meningococcus Typed by the polysaccharides of their capsules, and especially virulent in the tropics and in antibody-deficient patients.

Gonococcus IgA may block attachment to mucous surfaces, but the infection is seldom eliminated, leading to a 'carrier' state.

M. tuberculosis; leprosy These mycobacteria have very tough cell walls, rich in lipids, which resist intracellular killing; they also can inhibit phagosome-lysosome fusion. Chronic CMI results, with tissue destruction and scarring. In leprosy, a 'spectrum' between localisation and dissemination corresponds to a predominance of CMI and of antibody respectively.

Shigella and **Cholera** are confined to the intestine, and produce their effects by secreting exotoxins. However anti-toxin vaccines are much less effective than natural infection in inducing immunity.

Salmonella (e.g. **S. typhi**) infects the intestine but can also survive and spread within macrophages.

Tetanus owes its severity to the rapid action of its exotoxin on the CNS.

Diphtheria also secretes powerful neurotoxins, but death can be due to local tissue damage in the larynx ('false membrane').

Syphilis should be mentioned as an example of bacteria surviving all forms of immune attack without sheltering inside cells. Autoantibody to mitochondrial cardiolipin is the basis of the Wasserman Reaction. Cross-reactions of this type, due presumably to bacterial attempts to mimic host antigens and thus escape the attentions of the immune system, are clearly a problem to the host, who has to choose between ignoring the infection and making autoantibodies which may be damaging to his own tissues; see Fig 30 for a further discussion of Autoimmunity.

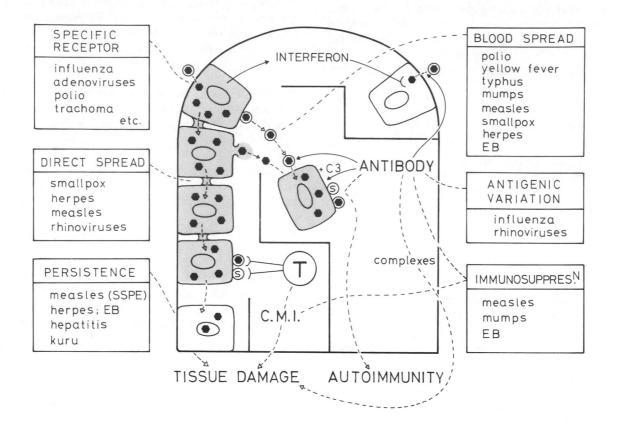

SPECIFIC RECEPTOR

influenza
adenoviruses
polio
trachoma
etc.

DIRECT SPREAD

smallpox
herpes
measles
rhinoviruses

PERSISTENCE

measles (SSPE)
herpes; EB
hepatitis
kuru

INTERFERON

ANTIBODY

+ C3

complexes

C.M.I.

BLOOD SPREAD

polio
yellow fever
typhus
mumps
measles
smallpox
herpes
EB

ANTIGENIC VARIATION

influenza
rhinoviruses

IMMUNOSUPPRES.N

measles
mumps
EB

TISSUE DAMAGE   AUTOIMMUNITY

Viruses (depicted here as black hexagons) differ from bacteria in lacking walls based on muramic acid and being unable to replicate outside the cells of their host. The key process in virus infection is therefore **intracellular replication** (shaded cells), which may or may not lead to cell death.

For rapid protection, **interferon** (top) plays the same 'natural antibiotic' role as lysozyme in bacterial infection, though the mechanism is quite different. Antibody (right) is valuable in preventing entry and blood-borne spread of some viruses, but the ability of others to spread from cell to cell (left) puts the burden of adaptive immunity on the T-cell system, which specialises in recognising altered 'self' histocompatibility antigens (**S**). Macrophages (not shown) may play a role as effectors in all three types of immunity. The antibody-forming system can also

respond to altered self, often producing anti-self (auto-) antibodies in the process (see Autoimmunity; Fig 30).

As with bacteria, some of the most virulent virus infections are zoonoses, e.g. rabies (dogs), yellow fever (monkeys). At the other end of the scale, some viruses can persist for years without symptoms, and then be reactivated to cause serious diseases, possibly including tumours.

Intermediate between viruses and bacteria are those obligatory intracellular organisms which do possess cell walls (Rickettsiae, Trachoma) and others without walls but capable of extracellular replication (Mycoplasma). Immunologically the former are closer to viruses, the latter to bacteria.

INTERFERON

A group of proteins (MW 20-160,000) produced in response to virus infection (and also DS-RNA, LPS, etc) which stimulates cells to make a protein that blocks viral mRNA transcription, and thus protects them from infection. It can be made by non-lymphoid (type I) and also lymphoid (T) cells (type 2). It has effects on normal cell division too and if available in large amounts might be useful as an anti-viral and perhaps anti-tumour agent.

T; C.M.I. As described in Figs 16 and 17, cytotoxic T cells 'learn' to recognise Class I MHC antigens, and then respond to these in association with virus antigens on the cell surface; since almost any type of cell can harbour viruses, it is appropriate that Class I MHC antigens are expressed on most cells (unlike, for example, Class II MHC antigens). It was during the study of antiviral immunity in mice that the vital role of the MHC in T-cell responses was discovered.

It is not known exactly how cytotoxic T cells kill their target, but it involves cell contact and has features suggesting 'induced suicide'.

VIRUSES

There is no proper taxonomy for viruses, which can be classified according to: size; the nature of their genome (DNA or RNA), how they spread (budding, cytolysis or directly; all are illustrated), and — of special interest here — whether they are eliminated or merely driven into hiding by the immune response. Brief details of some important viruses are given below.

Pox viruses (smallpox, vaccinia). Large; DNA; spread locally, avoiding antibody, as well as in blood leucocytes; express antigens on the infected cell, attracting C.M.I. The antigenic cross-reaction between these two viruses is the basis for the use of vaccinia to protect against smallpox (Jenner, 1798, but known in the Far East for thousands of years). Thanks to this vaccine, smallpox is the first disease ever to have been eliminated from the entire globe. Severe T-cell deficiency (see Fig 33) often presents as a progressive, fatal, inability to control vaccinia.

Herpes viruses (herpes simplex, varicella, EB (Epstein-Barr)). Medium; DNA; tend to persist and cause different symptoms when reactivated: thus varicella (chickenpox) reappears as zoster (shingles); EB (infectious mononucleosis) may initiate malignancy (Burkitt's lymphoma).

Viruses continued

Adenoviruses (influenza, mumps, measles). Large; RNA; spread by budding. Influenza is the classic example of attachment by specific receptor (haemagglutinin) and also of antigenic variation, which accounts for the relative uselessness of adaptive immunity. Mumps, by spreading in the testis, can initiate autoimmune damage. Measles infects lymphocytes, causes nonspecific suppression of CMI, and persists to cause SSPE (subacute sclerosing panencephalitis); some workers feel that multiple sclerosis may also be a disease of this type.

Arboviruses (Arthropod-Borne; yellow fever). Small; RNA. Blood spread to the liver leads to jaundice. Good immunity and protection by vaccine.

Polio virus Small; RNA. Only 'seen' by the immune system on entry (via the gut) and when the host cell is lysed, and therefore susceptible to antibody (including IgA) but not CMI.

Hepatitis can be caused by at least two viruses: A (infective) and B (serum-transmitted). In the latter, immune complexes and autoantibodies are found, and virus can persist in 'carriers', particularly in tropical countries.

Trachoma An organism of the Psittacosis group (Chlamydia). The frightful scarring of the conjunctiva may be due to over-vigorous CMI.

Typhus and other Rickettsiae may survive in macrophages, like the tubercle bacillus.

Kuru The most extreme example of a 'slow' virus, causing progressive brain damage and only spread by cannibalism.

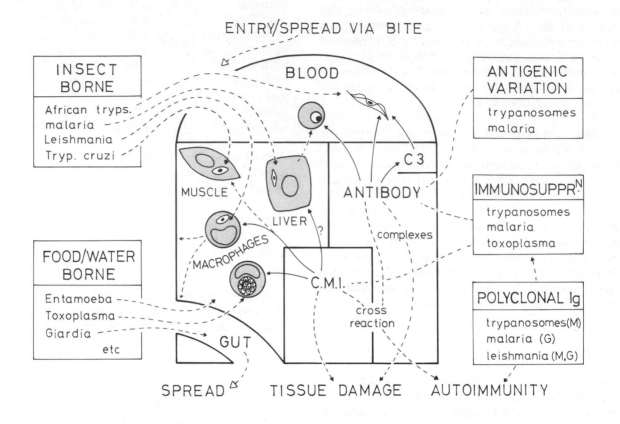

Relatively few (less than 20) protozoa infest man, but among these are four of the most formidable parasites of all, in terms of numbers affected and severity of disease: malaria, the African and American trypanosomes, and the Leishmanias (top left). These owe their success to combinations of strategy also found among bacteria and viruses — long-distance **spread** by insect vectors (cf. plague, typhus, yellow fever), **intracellular** habitat (shaded in the figure; cf. tuberculosis, viruses), **antigenic variation** (cf. influenza), **immunosuppression** (cf. measles) — but so highly developed that complete acquired resistance to protozoal infections is quite exceptional, and what immunity there is often serves merely to keep parasite numbers down ('premunition') and the host alive, to the advantage of the parasite. The rationale for vaccination is correspondingly weak, especially since some of the symptoms of these diseases appear to be due to the immune response rather than to the parasite itself.

By contrast, the intestinal protozoa (bottom left) generally cause fairly mild disease, except when immunity is deficient or suppressed. Micro-organisms which only cause trouble in immunodeficient patients are called 'opportunistic'; they include bacteria (Pseudomonas, Listeria), viruses (Cytomegalovirus, Zoster), and fungi (Candida) as well as protozoa (Pneumocystis, Toxoplasma), and their existence testifies to the unobtrusive efficiency of the normal immune system.

African trypanosomes *T. gambiense* and *T. rhodesiense*, carried by tsetse flies, cause sleeping sickness in West and East Africa respectively. The blood form, though susceptible to antibody and complement, survives by repeatedly replacing its surface coat of glycoprotein 'variant antigen' by a gene-switching mechanism; the number of variants is unknown but large (at least 25). High levels of non-specific IgM, including autoantibodies, coexist with suppressed antibody responses to other antigens such as vaccines; this may be due to polyclonal activation of B cells by a parasite product (cf. bacterial lipopolysaccharides).

Malaria *Plasmodium falciparum* (the most serious), *P. malariae*, *P. vivax* and *P. ovale* are transmitted by mosquitoes. There is a brief liver stage, against which vaccination can protect, possibly via cell-mediated immunity, followed by a cyclical invasion of red cells, against which antibody is partially effective; antigenic variation and polyclonal IgG production may account for the slow development of immunity. Vaccination protects against the red-cell stage in certain animal models. Human red cells lacking the Duffy blood group, or containing foetal haemoglobin, are 'naturally' resistant to *P. vivax* and *P. falciparum* respectively. *P. malariae* is specially prone to induce immune complex deposition in the kidney.

Leishmania a confusing variety of parasites, carried by sandflies, which cause an even more bewildering array of diseases in different parts of the tropics. The organisms inhabit macrophages, and the pathology (mainly in the skin and viscera) seems to depend on the strength of cell-mediated immunity and/or its balance with antibody (cf. leprosy). Cutaneous leishmaniasis in Africa is unusual in stimulating self-cure and subsequent resistance to the more serious visceral disease. This example of cross-protection has apparently been known and applied in the Middle East for many centuries.

Trypanosoma cruzi, the cause of Chagas' disease in Central and South America, is transmitted from animal reservoirs by reduviid bugs. It infects many cells, notably cardiac muscle and autonomic nervous ganglia. There is some suggestion that cell-mediated autoimmunity against normal cardiac muscle may be responsible for the chronic heart failure. The organism has been killed *in vitro* by antibody and eosinophils.

Toxoplasma *T. gondii* is particularly virulent in the foetus and immuno-suppressed patients, chiefly affecting the brain and eye. It can survive inside macrophages by preventing phagolysosome formation (cf. tuberculosis), but cell-mediated immunity can overcome this. Toxoplasma stimulates macrophages and suppresses T cells, leading to varied effects on resistance to other infections.

Entameoba histolytica normally causes disease in the colon (amoebic dysentery), but can get via the blood to the liver, brain, etc, and cause dangerous abscesses. Some animals, and perhaps man, develop a degree of immunity, of unknown type.

Giardia, Balantidium, Isospora etc normally restrict their effects to the gut causing dysentery and occasionally malabsorption.

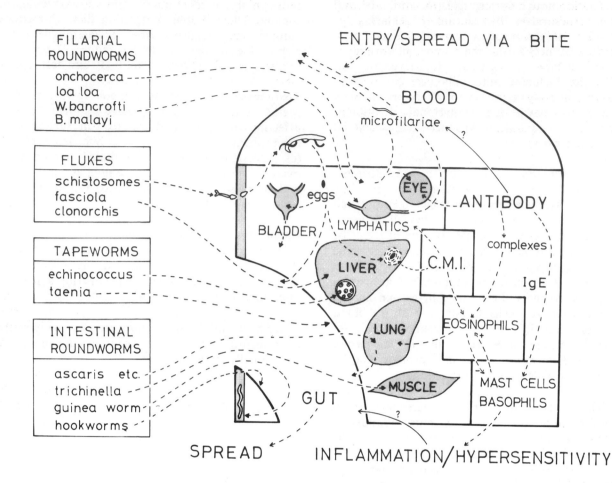

Parasitic worms of all three classes (roundworms, tapeworms, and flukes) are responsible for numerous human diseases, including three of the most unpleasant (upper left): Onchocerciasis, elephantiasis and Schistosomiasis. These worms are transmitted with the aid of specific insect or snail vectors, and are restricted to the tropics, while the remainder (lower left) can be picked up anywhere by eating food contaminated with their eggs, larvae, or cysts. A feature of many worm infections is their complex life cycles and circuitous migratory patterns, during which they often take up residence in a particular organ (shaded in figure).

Another striking feature is the predominance of **eosinophils** and of **IgE**; as a result, hypersensitivity reactions in skin, lung, etc, are common, but whether these are ever protective is still controversial. Since they do not replicate in the human host (unlike protozoa, bacteria and viruses), individual worms must resist the immune response particularly well in order to survive, and, as with the best-adapted protozoa (cf. malaria), immunity operates, if at all, to keep down the numbers of worms rather than to eliminate them. The outlook for vaccination might seem very dim, but it is surprisingly effective in certain dog and cattle infections.

Mystifying, but provocative, is the finding that several drugs originally used against worms (Niridazole, Levamisole, Hetrazan) turn out to have suppressive or stimulatory effects on T cells, inflammation, and other immunological elements.

Eosinophils may have three effects in worm infections: phagocytosis of the copious antigen-antibody complexes, modulation of hypersensitivity by inactivation of mediators, and (*in vitro*, at least) killing of certain worms with the aid of IgG antibody. Eosinophilia is partly due to mast cell and T cell chemotactic factors; T cells may also stimulate output.

IgE Worms, and even some worm extracts, stimulate specific and non-specific IgE production; it has been suggested but not proved that the resulting inflammatory response (e.g. in the gut) may hinder worm attachment or entry. There is also a belief that the high IgE levels, by blocking mast cells, can prevent allergy to pollen etc.

ROUNDWORMS (Nematodes) may be Filarial (in which the first-stage larva, or microfiliaria, can only develop in an insect, and only the third stage is infective to man), or Intestinal (in which full development can occur in the patient).

Filarial Nematodes

Onchocerca volvulus is spread by Simulium flies, which deposit larvae and collect microfilariae in the skin. Microfilaria also inhabit the eye, causing 'river blindness' which may be largely due to immune responses. In the Middle East, pathology is restricted to the skin; parasitologists and immunologists disagree as to whether this reflects different species or a disease spectrum (cf. leprosy). *Loa loa* (loasis) is somewhat similar but less severe.
W. (Wuchereria) bancrofti and *B. (Brugia) malayi* are spread by mosquitoes, which suck microfilariae from the blood. The larvae inhabit lymphatics, causing elephantiasis, partly by blockage and partly by inducing cell-mediated immune responses; soil elements (e.g. silicates) may also be involved. In some animal models, microfilaraemia can be controlled by antibody.

Intestinal Nematodes

Ascaris, Strongyloides, Toxocara Travelling through the lung, larvae may cause asthma, etc, associated with eosinophilia. *Trichinella spiralis* larvae encyst in muscles. In some animal models, worms of this type stimulate good protective immunity.

Guinea worms (Dracunculus) live under the skin and can be up to 4 feet long. **Hookworms** (Ancylostoma, Necator) enter through the skin and live in the small intestine on blood, causing severe anaemia. None of these worms appear to stimulate useful immunity.

FLUKES (Trematodes) spend part of their life cycle in a snail, from which the cercariae infect man either by penetrating the skin (**Schistosomes**) or by being eaten (**Fasciola, Clonorchis**). The latter ('liver flukes') inhabit the liver but do not induce protective immunity.

Schistosomes ('blood flukes') live and mate harmlessly in venous blood (*S.mansoni, S.japonicum*: mesenteric; *S.haematobium*: bladder), only causing trouble when their eggs are trapped in the liver or bladder, where strong granulomatous T-cell mediated reactions lead to fibrosis in the liver and nodules and sometimes cancer in the bladder. The adult worms evade immune attack by covering their surface with antigens derived from host cells, at the same time stimulating antibody which may destroy subsequent infections at an early stage ('concomitant immunity'). Eosinophils, macrophages, IgG, and IgE have all been implicated.

TAPEWORMS (Cestodes) may live harmlessly in the intestine (e.g. **Taenia**), occasionally invading, and dying in, the brain ('cysticercosis'), or establish cystic colonies in the liver etc (e.g. the hydatid cysts of **Echinococcus**), where the worms are shielded from the effects of antibody.

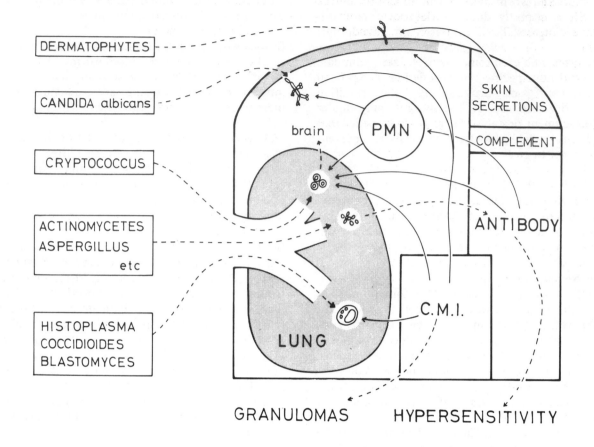

Fungal infections are normally only a superficial nuisance (e.g. ringworm: top), but a few fungi can cause serious systemic disease, usually entering via the lung in the form of spores (centre left); the outcome depends on the degree and type of immune response, and may range from an unnoticed respiratory episode to rapid fatal dissemination or a violent hypersensitivity reaction.

In general, the survival mechanisms of successful fungi are similar to those of bacteria: anti-phagocytic capsules (e.g. cryptococcus), resistance to digestion within macrophages (e.g. histoplasma etc), and destruction of polymorphs (e.g. coccidiodes). Some yeasts activate complement via the alternative pathway, but it is not known if this has any effect on survival.

Perhaps the most interesting fungus from the immunological point of view is *Candida albicans* (upper left), a common and harmless inhabitant of skin and mucous membranes which readily takes advantage of any weakening of host resistance. This is most strikingly seen when polymorphs (PMN) or T cells are defective, but it also occurs in patients who are undernourished, immunosuppressed, iron deficient, alcoholic, diabetic, aged, or simply 'run down' (see Immunodeficiency Fig 33).

PMN Polymorphonuclear leucocyte ('neutrophil'), an important phagocytic cell. Recurrent fungal as well as bacterial infections may be due to defects in PMN numbers or function, which may in turn be genetic or drug-induced (steroids, antibiotics). Functional defects may affect chemotaxis ('lazy leucocyte'), phago-lysosome formation (Chediak-Higashi syndrome), peroxide production (Chronic Granulomatous Disease), myeloperoxidase, and other enzymes. Deficiencies in complement or antibody will of course also compromise phagocytosis.

Dermatophytes filamentous fungi which metabolise keratin and therefore live off skin, hair, and nails (ringworm). Sebaceous secretions help to control them, but CMI may also play an ill-defined part.

Candida albicans (Monilia); a yeast-like fungus which causes severe spreading infections of the skin, mouth, etc in patients with immunodeficiency, especially T-cell defects. Remarkable clinical improvement, together which restoration of a positive delayed hypersensitivity skin test, has been induced by 'Transfer Factor', an extract of normal leucocytes originally believed to confer specific T-cell responsive-ness but now thought to be non-antigen-specific, albeit effective. The precise role of T cells in controlling this infection is not understood.

Cryptococcus a capsulated yeast able to resist phagocytosis unless opsonised by antibody and/or complement (cf. pneumococcus etc). In immunodeficient patients, spread to the brain and meninges is a serious complication.

Actinomycetes and other sporing fungi from mouldy hay etc. can reach the lung alveoli, stimulate antibody production, and subsequently induce severe hypersensitivity ('farmer's lung'). Both IgG and IgE may be involved. **Aspergillus** is particularly prone to cause trouble in patients with tuberculosis.

Histoplasma (Histoplasmosis), **Coccidiodes** (Coccidio-mycosis), and **Blastomyces** (Blastomycosis) are similar in causing pulmonary disease, particularly in America, which may either heal spontaneously, disseminate body-wide, or progress to chronic granulomatosis and fibrosis, depending on the immunological status of the patient. The obvious resemblance to tuberculosis and leprosy emphasises the point that it is microbial survival mechanisms (in this case, resistance to digestion in macrophages) rather than taxonomic relationships, which determine the pattern of disease.

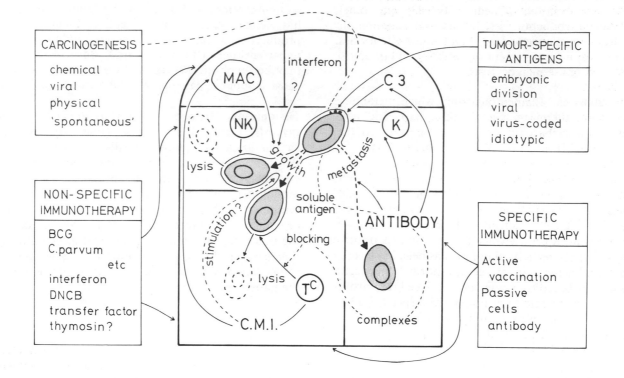

Immunologists like to feel that when the 'conquest of cancer' is announced they will be among those sharing the credit, but it must be admitted that on present evidence this cannot be guaranteed. In its relationship to the host, a tumour cell (shaded in figure) is rather like a successful parasite, with special additional features. Parasite-like mechanisms that may help prevent elimination include: **weak antigenicity** and extensive cross-reaction with self; **immunosuppression**; release of **soluble antigens**; antigen-antibody **complexes**; and **antigenic variation**. Unlike parasites, however, spontaneous tumours are unique and usually of unknown origin, and they unfortunately lack the well-adapted parasite's sense of self-preservation through host-preservation, (behaving more like virulent zoonoses). Moreover, apart from some childhood tumours, cancer occurs at too late an age to have had much selective effect on the evolution of immune defences.

Nevertheless there are hopeful pointers. Most tumour cells *are* antigenic (top right), albeit weakly, and experimental animals can often be specifically immunised against them. Immunodeficient and immunosuppressed patients do develop more tumours of certain tissues (though T-cell deprived mice do not). Cells that kill tumours *in vitro*, and rejection of secondary implants ('concomitant immunity'), can be found in animals with growing primary tumours. Most encouraging of all, tumours occasionally regress spontaneously, or after only partial destruction by surgery or chemotherapy.

As to which immune mechanisms (solid lines and arrows) are, or might be made, effective, opinion has swung away from all-embracing theories such as 'T-cell surveillance' (which was an attempt to rationalise transplant rejection) towards the concept that different mechanisms, both natural (top) and adaptive (bottom), may work against different tumours — as they do against different infectious micro-organisms.

CARCINOGENESIS
TUMOUR ANTIGENS

In mice, chemicals such as methylcholanthrene, benzpyrenes, etc tend to induce tumours each with unique **'idiotypic'** antigens, whilst tumours induced by viruses, such as Polyoma, Gross leukaemia, etc., share antigens characteristic of the virus. Either type may be able to immunise against subsequent challenge, in which case they are called 'tumour-specific transplantation antigens' (TSTA). In man, only the Epstein-Barr (EB) virus is linked to tumour development, but antigen-sharing, perhaps a sign of viral origin, is found among neuroblastomas and osteosarcomas.

Embryonic antigens absent from normal adult cells may be re-expressed when they become malignant. Carcino-embryonic antigen (CEA) in the colon and α-foetoprotein in the liver are examples, of diagnostic value.

Division antigens, and antigens characteristic of one **stage** of cell maturation, may be common in tumours and extremely rare in normal tissues; an example is the 'stem-cell' antigen of acute lymphoblastic leukaemia.

NATURAL IMMUNITY

Mac macrophages, especially when activated, can prevent growth of some tumours *in vitro* without killing them ('cytostasis'). **Interferon** may possibly do the same. In the absence of evidence that either can recognise malignancy *per se*, this is presumed to reflect some kind of general growth-controlling function. But in experimental animals it has been shown that extreme macrophage activation can result in the release of factors that actually kill some tumours *in vivo* ('tumour necrotic factors'). Which of the dozens of lysosomal and other macrophage products these are is still uncertain.

NK 'Natural killer' cell, a small lymphocyte-like cell of unknown origin, which can lyse certain tumour cells *in vitro*, apparently unaided by antibody.

K 'Killer' cell, another small cell found in blood, marrow, etc, as part of the 'null' (i.e. not obviously T or B) lymphocyte population, but probably belonging to the myeloid lineage. It can kill tumour cells coated with IgG antibody, without phagocytosis.

C3 The third component of complement can apparently be activated by some tumour cell surfaces via the alternative pathway. This and the three above mechanisms may contribute to the surprising resistance of thymusless 'nude' mice to spontaneous tumours.

Antibody As with micro-organisms, antibody is more likely to be effective against free cells (leukaemia; metastasising tumours) than those in solid lumps. However it can also 'enhance' tumour growth, probably by forming complexes with soluble antigens and blocking T-cell-mediated cytotoxicity. An interesting antibody is found in patients with Burkitt's lymphoma and also in Infectious Mononucleosis, a benign disease caused by the EB virus; it has been suggested that immunodeficiency due to malaria may explain the different course of disease in the tropics, where progression to Burkitt's lymphoma is common.

Cell-mediated immunity Cytotoxic T cells can often be demonstrated *in vitro*, and in mice they can sometimes eliminate a tumour *in vivo*. T cells can activate macrophages. But there is also a theory that weak T cell reactions can actually stimulate tumour growth.

NON-SPECIFIC IMMUNOTHERAPY

BCG (an attenuated tubercle bacillus) and **Corynebacterium parvum** have been tried against melanoma, sarcoma, etc, especially combined with other treatments. Their major immunological effect seems to be macrophage activation, but they may also affect NK cells. A tremendous range of bacterial and other immunostimulating agents is at present being tested for anti-tumour activity (see Fig 34).

DNCB (dinitrochlorobenzene), a strong inducer of delayed hypersensitivity, has been used to non-specifically damage local skin tumours, while to improve T-cell reactivity in general, transfer factor, thymosin, and various drugs (e.g. levamisole) have their advocates.

SPECIFIC IMMUNOTHERAPY

Vaccination with irradiated or enzyme-treated cells, cell hybrids, etc can be very successful in animals before tumour induction, but may also be of benefit in patients after chemotherapy or surgery.

Passive antibody might theoretically be able to remove blocking antigen and facilitate T-cell function. Cells primed against the patient's own tumour have also been tried, but of course they have to come from animals and there is the problem of rejection. However cancer is a desperate situation and desperate remedies may be better than none.

26 Harmful immunity: A general scheme

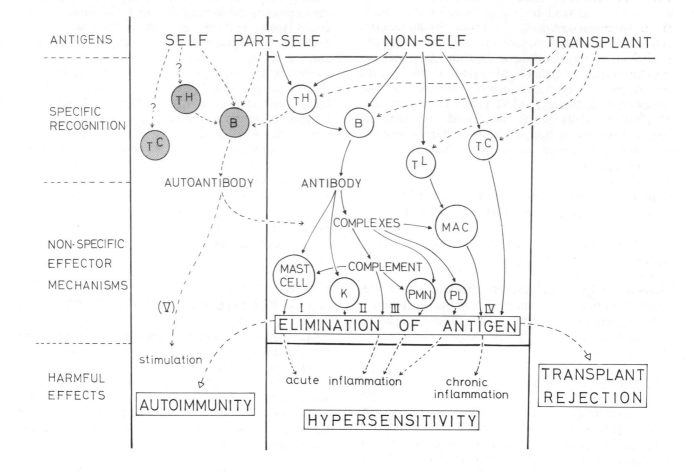

The immune system owes its success against microbial infection to two characteristic properties: the wide range of antigens it can specifically recognise, and the strong non-specific effector mechanisms it can mobilise to eliminate them. Unfortunately both properties can also operate against their possessor. (1) Wide-ranging specificity necessitates an efficient mechanism for avoiding action against 'self' determinants and for deciding whether or not to act against targets that are part-self and part non-self (top left), which includes several extracellular and all intracellular micro-organisms (the problem of **Autoimmunity**). Also there are cases where the elimination of non-self material may not be desirable (the problem of **Transplant Rejection**; right). (2) Strong non-specific weapons (e.g. complement, polymorphs, macrophages, and other inflammatory agents: lower centre) cannot always be trained precisely on the proper target, but may spill over to damage neighbouring tissues (the problem of **Hypersensitivity**).

The nomenclature of these **immunopathological** reactions has never been very tidy. Originally any evidence of altered reactivity to an antigen following prior contact was called 'Allergy', while 'Hypersensitivity', though intended for those effects which harmed the host, was in fact defined as 'acute', 'immediate', or 'delayed' on the basis of the time taken for changes — often quite innocuous skin test reactions — to appear. As knowledge grew, reactions could be classified according to mechanism; this is the basis of the very influential scheme of Gell and Coombs (Types I to IV; lower centre), in which 'Allergy' and 'Hypersensitivity' retained their old meaning, but with the latter extended to include autoimmunity and transplant rejection. However most immunologists now use 'Allergy' in its everyday sense of immediate (Type I) hypersensitivity, e.g. to pollen. What is really needed is a separate word*, without historical overtones, to cover those aspects for which specific recognition is not to blame (that is, excluding autoimmunity and transplant rejection). Meanwhile, it is safest to think in terms of both specific recognition *and* effector mechanisms when considering immunologically-mediated tissue damage.

* Some recommend 'indirect'; I like 'immunoflammatory'.

26

T^{**H**} Helper T cell, whose recognition of carrier determinants permits antibody responses by B cells. There is little evidence that helper T cells ever react to unaltered 'self' antigens *in vivo*.

B B lymphocyte, the potentially antibody-forming cell. B lymphocytes that recognise many, though probably not all, 'self' determinants are found in normal animals (shaded in the Figure); they can be switched on to make autoantibody by 'part-self' (or 'cross-reacting') antigens if a helper T cell can recognise a 'non-self' determinant on the same antigen (e.g. a drug or a virus; for further details see Fig 30).

T^{**C**} Cytotoxic T cell, able to kill allogeneic or 'altered-self' targets. Cytotoxicity against 'pure' self may occur *in vitro* but has never been clearly shown *in vivo*, perhaps because it is so easily blocked.

T^{**L**} The lymphokine-secreting cell responsible for attracting and activating macrophages etc. Autoreactivity has not been proved here either.

Mast cell A tissue cell with basophilic granules containing vasoactive amines, etc, which can be released following interaction of antigen with passively-acquired surface antibody (IgE), resulting in rapid inflammation, local ('allergy') or systemic ('anaphylaxis').

K 'Killer' cell; a lymphocyte-like cell capable of killing antibody (IgG) coated cells *in vitro*. It may be involved in some autoimmune and transplantation reactions, but has not been incriminated in 'immunoflammation'.

Complexes Combination with antigen is, of course, the basis of all effects of antibody. It is when the resulting complex is not phagocytosed, but instead circulates in 'soluble' form, that tissue damage may occur from the activation of complement, PMN, or platelets.

Complement is responsible for many of the tissue-damaging effects of antigen-antibody interactions, as well as their useful function against micro-organisms. The 'immunoflammatory' effects are mostly due to the anaphylotoxins (C3a and C5a) which act on mast cells, while opsonisation (by C3b) and lysis (by C5-9) are important in the destruction of transplanted cells and (via autoantibody) of autoantigens.

PMN Polymorphonuclear leucocytes are attracted rapidly to sites of inflammation by complement-mediated chemotaxis, where they phagocytose antigen-antibody complexes; their lysosomal enzymes can cause tissue destruction, as in the classic Arthus reaction.

PL Platelets. Antigen-antibody complexes bind to and aggregate platelets, causing vascular obstruction as well as vasoactive amine release. Platelet aggregation is a prominent feature of kidney graft rejection.

MAC Macrophages are important in phagocytosis, but may also be attracted and activated, largely by T cells, to the site of antigen persistence, resulting in both tissue necrosis and granuloma formation. The slower arrival of monocytes and macrophages in the skin following antigen injection gave rise to the name 'delayed hypersensitivity'.

TYPES OF HYPERSENSITIVITY:
(Gell and Coombs classification)

I. Acute (anaphylactic; immediate; reaginic): Mediated by IgE, and sometimes IgG, antibody together with mast cells. Example: hay fever.
II. Antibody-mediated (cytotoxic): mediated by IgG or IgM together with complement, K cells, or phagocytic cells. Examples: blood transfusion reactions; many autoimmune diseases. (Not true immunoflammation).
III. Complex-mediated: inflammation involving complement, polymorphs, etc. Examples: Arthus reaction; serum sickness; chronic glomerulonephritis.
IV. Cell-mediated (delayed; tuberculin-type): T-cell dependent recruitment of macrophages, eosinophils, etc. Examples: tuberculoid leprosy; schistosomal cirrhosis; viral skin rashes; skin graft rejection.
V. Stimulatory: a recent proposal to split off from Type II those cases where antibody directly stimulates a cell function. Example: stimulation of the thyroid TSH receptor in thyrotoxicosis. For the sake of completeness, a place must also be found somewhere for the 'blocking' and 'enhancing' antibodies of tumour immunity, and for polyclonal B cell activation (e.g. in trypanosomiasis), both of which can be against the patient's best interests.

27 Anaphylaxis and allergy

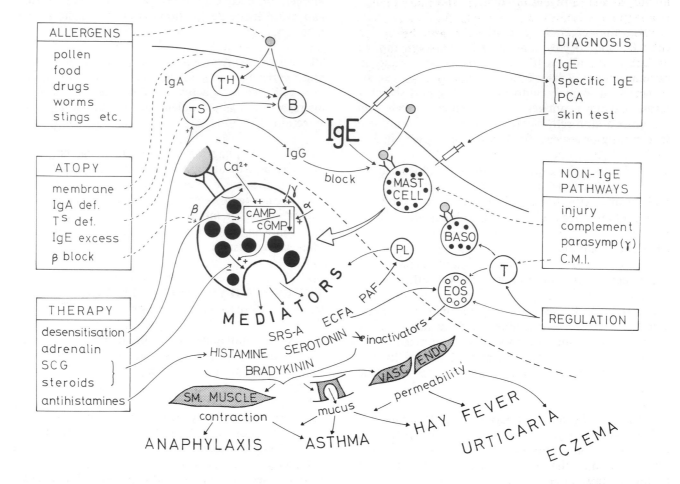

Anaphylaxis, or 'anaphylactic shock', a rare but terrifying response to penicillin, bee stings etc; and hay fever, so common (more than one person in ten) as to be almost normal, are both caused by the same basic process: the production of **IgE** antibody (top centre), its attachment to **mast cells** (centre) and, on renewed contact with the same antigen, explosive degranulation of the mast cells and release of **mediators** (lower centre) which act on smooth muscle, mucous glands, and blood vessels. With massive release (anaphylaxis) there is bronchospasm, vomiting, skin rashes, oedema of the nose and throat, and vascular collapse, sometimes fatal, whilst with more localised release one or other of these symptoms predominates, depending on the site of exposure to the antigen.

Antigens that can trigger these reactions are known as 'allergens' (top left; shaded circles); they have very diverse origins but a curious similarity of molecular weight (20,000-40,000). People who suffer unduly from allergy are called 'atopic'; this trait is usually inherited and has been attributed to a variety of constitutional abnormalities (centre left). To justify the existence of this unpleasant and apparently useless form of immune response, it has been assumed to date from a time when worm infections (or perhaps insect bites!) were a serious evolutionary threat. Inflammation itself, of course, is an invaluable part of the response to injury and infection, and where injury is minimal (e.g. worms in the gut), IgE offers a rapid and specific trigger for increasing access of blood cells etc, to the area.

There is a close link between inflammation and the emotions via the autonomic nervous system, through the influence of the sympathetic (α and β) and parasympathetic (γ) receptors on intracellular levels of cyclic nucleotides, which in turn regulate cell function — in the case of mast cells, mediator release. Note also that mast cell degranulation can be triggered directly by tissue injury (see Fig 6) and complement activation (see Fig 28).

27

IgE The major class of reaginic (skin sensitising; homocytotropic) antibody. Normally less than 1/10,000 of total Ig, its level can be up to 30 times higher, and specific antibody levels 100 times higher, in allergic or worm-infested patients. Binding of its Fc portion to receptors on mast cells and basophils, followed by cross-linking of adjacent molecules by antigen, triggers degranulation. Antigen-responsiveness can be transferred to guinea-pigs by serum — the Passive Cutaneous Anaphylaxis (PCA) test.

IgA antibody normally protects skin and mucous surfaces, and deficiency of IgA is thought to facilitate entry of antigens and stimulation of IgE.

IgG antibody, by efficiently removing antigens, can protect against mast cell degranulation. However some IgG subclasses (in the human, IgG4) may have transient reagenic effects as well.

T^H Helper T cell. IgE production by B cells is highly T-cell dependent.

T^S Suppressor T cell. IgE is also very sensitive to suppression, which may, together with IgG production, account for the success of 'desensitisation' by specific antigen injections.

Mast cells and blood **Basophils** are broadly similar, but there are differences in mediator content and the effect of drugs.

PL Platelets contain many of the same mediators as mast cells, but IgE is not directly responsible for their release.

EOS Eosinophils are attracted by the mast-cell product **ECF** (Eosinophil chemotactic factor) **A**, and release enzymes that neutralise the inflammatory mediators. They thus play an important part in homeostasis.

T T cells. Attraction and stimulation of basophils and eosinophils occurs as part of 'cell-mediated' (Type IV) reactions, presumably to expedite and control them.

Ca^{2+} The entry of calcium ions is thought to be the first consequence of IgE cross-linking at the mast-cell surface.

cAMP, cGMP cyclic adenosine/guanosine monophosphate, the relative levels of which regulate cell activity. A fall in the cAMP/cGMP ratio is favoured by Ca^{2+} entry and by activation of α and γ receptors, and results in degranulation. Activation of the β receptor (e.g. by adrenalin) has the opposite effect; atopic patients may have a partial defect of β receptor function, permitting excessive mediator release.

MEDIATORS

Histamine has a rapid, and **Bradykinin** and **SRS** (slow-reacting substance) **A** a slower contracting effect on smooth muscle; histamine and bradykinin and, in some animals, serotonin also affect the **vascular endothelium** and **mucus** secretion. Mast cells also contain heparin, but this has no known function in inflammation.

PAF Platelet Aggregating Factor promotes the release of histamine by platelets.

ECF-A Eosinophil Chemotactic Factor (see above).

SCG Sodium chromoglycate ('Intal'), and **steroids** (e.g. betamethasone) are thought to inhibit mediator release by stabilising lysosomal membranes. Other drugs used in allergy include **antihistamines** (which do not, however, counteract the other mediators), **adrenalin**, isoprenaline, etc, which stimulate β receptors, anti-cholinergics (e.g. atropine), which block γ receptors, and theophylline, which raises cAMP levels. It has been gratifying to physicians to see the new molecular pharmacology of cell regulation confirming so many of their empirical observations on the control of allergic disease.

ALLERGIC DISEASES

Originally the term 'atopy' referred only to hay fever and asthma, which are usually due to plant or animal 'allergens' in the air, such as pollens, fungi, and mites; it is still debatable whether all asthma is caused by allergy. However similar allergens may also cause skin reactions (urticaria), either from local contact or following absorption. Urticaria after eating shellfish, strawberries, cow's milk, etc is a clear case where the site of entry and the site of reaction are quite different, due to the ability of IgE antibodies to attach to mast cells anywhere in the body. There is mounting evidence for the role of food allergy in migraine and in other ill-defined physical and mental 'aches and pains'.

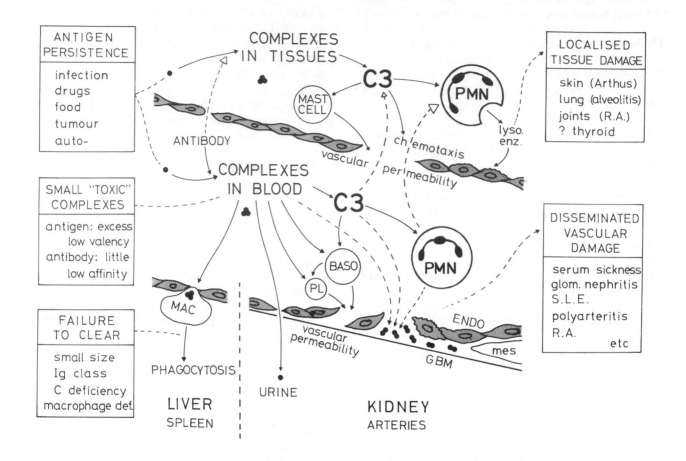

Less acute than the reactions mediated by IgE and mast cells (hours, days, or weeks rather than minutes) are the inflammatory responses caused by **antigen-antibody complexes** (black circles in figure); here **complement** (C3) and **polymorphonuclear leucocytes** (PMN) are the key agents of destruction. Normally, of course, complex formation is the prelude to disposal of antigen, but there are circumstances in which this fails to happen, chiefly because of the size of the complexes. Generally speaking, large complexes of the type that would precipitate *in vitro* are rapidly cleared by macrophages (lower left) especially in the liver (although if precipitation actually occurs in the tissues, inflammation may precede phagocytosis), whilst very small complexes may possibly pass harmlessly through the glomerulus into the urine; it is the ones formed in moderate antigen excess, with proportions such as Ag_3Ab_2 etc; which tend to stick in the walls of blood vessels, especially under the glomerular capillary endothelium (lower right), where they attract and activate complement and PMN, resulting in vascular damage. Complexes of this size are favoured by low antigen valency, and by low amounts or low affinity of antibody.

The resulting symptoms depend on whether the damage occurs locally in the tissues (top) or throughout the vascular system (centre), and also on whether exposure to the offending antigen is brief or repeated. Persistent exposure, as in chronic infections and even more when the antigen is a 'self' component (i.e. autoimmunity), is probably the commonest cause of chronic glomerulonephritis, itself the most frequent cause of renal failure.

Note that increased vascular permeability plays a preparatory role both for complex deposition in vessels and for exudation of complement and PMN into the tissues, underlining the close links between 'Type I' and 'Type III' immunoflammation. Note also that complement activation on a large enough scale can cause acute widespread vascular damage, with both clotting and haemorrhage; this serious complication of bacterial and viral diseases is known by several imposing names (Diffuse Intravascular Coagulation; Massive Complement Activation; and, when caused by bacterial endotoxin, Generalised Schwartzmann Reaction).

Complexes of small size are formed in antigen excess, as occurs early in the antibody response to a large dose of antigen, or with persistent exposure due to drugs, chronic infections (e.g. streptococci, hepatitis, malaria), or associated with autoantibodies.

MAC Macrophages lining the liver (Kuppfer cells) or spleen sinusoids remove particles from the blood, including large complexes.

PMN Polymorphonuclear leucocyte, the principal phagocyte of blood, whose granules (lysosomes) contain numerous antibacterial enzymes (**lyso. enz.**). When these are released, neighbouring cells are often damaged.

C3 The central component of complement, a series of serum proteins involved in inflammation and antibacterial immunity. C3 is split when complexes bind C1, C4, and C2, into a small fragment, C3a, which activates mast cells, and a larger one, C3b, which promotes phagocytosis by attaching to receptors on PMN (and macrophages). Subsequent components generate chemotactic factors that attract PMN to the site. C3 can also be split via the 'alternative' pathway initiated by bacterial endotoxins, etc.

Mast cells, **baso**phils, and **pl**atelets contribute to increased vascular permeability by releasing histamine etc.

GBM Glomerular basement membrane, which together with endothelial cells (**Endo.**) and external podocytes (not shown) separate blood from urine. Immune complexes are usually trapped on the blood side of the BM, except when antibody is specifically directed against the GBM itself, as in the autoimmune disease Goodpasture's Syndrome.

Mes mesangial cells, which proliferate into the subendothelial space, presumably in an attempt to remove complexes. Endothelial proliferation may occur too, resulting in glomerular thickening and loss of function.

The classic types of immune complex disease, neither of which is much seen nowadays, are the **Arthus Reaction**, in which antigen injected into the skin of animals with high levels of antibody induces local tissue necrosis, and **Serum Sickness**, in which passively injected (anti-) serum induces an antibody response early in the course of which small complexes are deposited in various blood vessels, causing a fever with skin and joint symptoms about a week later. Certain diseases, however, are thought to represent esentially the same type of pathological reactions.

SLE Systemic Lupus Erythematosus, a disease of unknown, possibly viral, origin in which autoantibodies to DNA and RNA are deposited, with complement, in the kidney, skin, joints, brain, etc. Treatment is by immunosuppression or, in severe cases, exchange transfusion to deplete autoantibody.

Polyarteritis nodosa; a disease of small arteries affecting numerous organs. Some cases may be due to complexes of Hepatitis B antigen with antibody and complement.

RA Rheumatoid arthritis features both local (Arthus-type) damage to joint surfaces and systemic vasculitis. The cause is unknown but autoantibodies to IgG are a constant finding.

Alveolitis caused by Actinomyces and other fungi (see Fig 24) may be due to an Arthus-type reaction in the lung.

Thyroiditis and perhaps other autoimmune diseases may be due to complex-mediated (i.e. autoantigen plus autoantibody) damage to the organ. With developments in the technique of detecting immune complexes (there are now over twenty different methods) it is likely that more diseases will be added to this list.

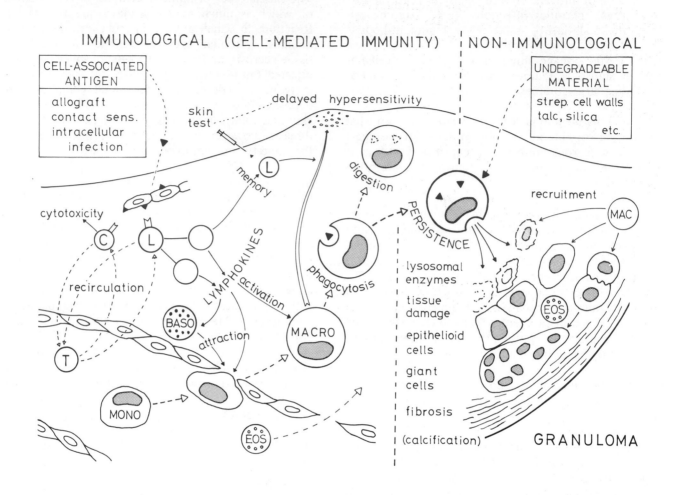

Following the changes in permeability, the activation of complement, and the influx of polymorphs, the last arrivals at sites of inflammation are the 'mononuclear cells': **lymphocytes** and **monocytes** (bottom left) Lymphocytes are usually specific in their attack, and only cause harm when attack is not called for (i.e. when the target is 'self' or a transplant), but monocytes and macrophages (the tissue form) are equipped with enzymes which they normally use in the process of mopping up dead tissue cells and polymorphs, but which can also damage healthy cells, including other macrophages. When the stimulus is persistent, the result may be a growing mass of macrophages, or granuloma (bottom right), the hallmark of **chronic inflammation**.

These changes can occur in the absence of any specific immune response (e.g. reactions to foreign bodies; top right), but they are often greatly augmented by the activity of specific T lymphocytes (left) which, by secreting lymphokines, attract and immobilise monocytes and activate macrophages. When this process is predominantly beneficial (as in healed tuberculosis) we speak of **'cell-mediated immunity'**; when it is harmful (as in contact sensitivity or schistosomal cirrhosis) it is termed **'Type IV hypersensitivity'**, the underlying pathology being the same and the difference one of emphasis (compare with Fig 16). Confusingly, direct killing by cytotoxic T cells is also called 'cell-mediated immunity', though since it mainly affects virus-containing cells, a better name would be 'cell-mediated autoimmunity' or, in the case of organ grafts, 'cell-mediated transplant rejection'.

In any case, it is rare for one type of tissue damage to occur in isolation, interacton of cells and sharing of biochemical pathways being a feature of immune mechanisms, useful and harmful alike.

CELL-MEDIATED IMMUNITY
(see Fig 16 for further details)

Contact between recirculating T cells and antigen leads to lymphokine secretion and effects on monocytes and other myeloid cells. The key feature is specific memory, which can be demonstrated *in vivo* by skin testing or *in vitro* by measuring the release of lymphokines such as MIF.

Chronic inflammation is tyical of persistent intracellular infections such as tuberculosis, leprosy, brucellosis, leishmaniasis, schistosomiasis (the egg granuloma), trichinosis, and fungi such as Histoplasma. See Figs 19-23 for further details.

CHRONIC NON-IMMUNOLOGICAL INFLAMMATION

Materials which are phagocytosed but cannot be degraded, or which are toxic to macrophages, such as talc, silica, asbestos, cotton wool, some metals and their salts, and bacterial products such as the cell wall peptidoglycan of group A streptococci, will give rise to granulomas even in T-cell deprived animals, and are therefore considered to be able to activate (or 'anger') macrophages without the aid of T cells.

GRANULOMAS are initiated and maintained by the recruitment of macrophages into the site where persistent antigen or toxic materials occur. Immune complexes are also a stimulus for granuloma formation.

Lysosomal enzymes, such as collagenase, elastase, cathepsins, etc, are released by macrophages and damage many normal tissue components.

Epithelioid cells are large cells found in palisades around necrotic tissue. They are thought to derive from macrophages, specialised for enzyme secretion rather than phagocytosis. There is some evidence that cell-mediated immunity favours their development.

Giant cells are formed by fusion of macrophages; they are particularly prominent in 'foreign-body granulomas.

Eosinophils are often found in granulomas, perhaps attracted by antigen-antibody complexes, but also under the influence of T cells. As in allergy (see Fig 26) their role may be regulatory.

Fibrosis around a granuloma represents an attempt at 'healing'. Long-standing granulomas, i.e. healed tuberculosis, may eventually calcify.

GRANULOMATOUS DISEASES

Apart from the known causes, granulomas are found in several disease of unknown aetiology, suggesting an irritant or immunological origin. A few of the better-known are listed below:

Sarcoidosis is characterised by nodules in the lung, skin, eye, etc. An interesting feature is a profound deficiency of T cell immunity and often an increased Ig level and antibody responsiveness.

Crohn's disease (regional ileitis) is somewhat like sarcoidosis, but usually restricted to the intestine. It has been claimed that it is due to autoimmunity against gut antigens stimulated by cross-reacting bacteria. **Ulcerative colitis** may have a similar aetiology.

Temporal arteritis is a chronic inflammatory disease of arteries, with granulomas in which giant cells are prominent.

30 Autoimmunity

ANTIGEN	ALTERED SELF				NORMAL SELF		
	altered MHC	drugs & infection		cross-reacting	sequestered	non-specific activation	B-cell mutation
EXAMPLE	viruses pox herpes E.B.	sedormid penicillin stibophen etc. ? malaria	α methyl dopa procainamide hydrallazine / virus mycoplasma	strep. A E.coli syphilis / hetero-antigens	lens sperm	adjuvants bacteria / G.V.H.	?
RECOGNITION / T CELLS / B CELLS	MHC, TC	S, TH, B	S, TH, TS, B	S, TH, TS, B	S, TC, TH, TS, B	S, TC, TH, TS, B	S, B
RESPONSE	cytotoxicity	antibody	antibody	antibody	?cytotox. antibody	?cytotox. antibody	antibody (monoclonal)
SPECIFICITY	altered self	non-self	self	self	self	self	self
EFFECT	1. elimination of virus 2. tissue damage	1. cell destruction (RBC, platelets, thyroid, stomach, adrenal, etc.) 2. interference with function (I.F., neuro-musc., sperm, thyroid) 3. immune complex disease (S.L.E., R.A., thyroid)					
	1	2	3	4	5	6	7

Autoimmunity is the mirror image of tolerance, reflecting the *loss* of tolerance to 'self', and before proceeding, the reader is recommended to glance back at Fig 18, which summarises the mechanisms by which the immune system normally safeguards its lymphocytes against self-reactivity.

The lymphocytes most prone to self-reactivity are cytotoxic T cells and B cells. Two situations need to be distinguished: (a) the destruction of **'altered-self'** cells, which is part of the normal activity of T cells against viruses (column 1), but which may also result from antibody formation against foreign materials that attach to cell surfaces (column 2), and (b) attack against perfectly **normal** cells or molecules because their antigens have unexpectedly stimulated a response. In the latter case (columns 3-6), antibody is predominantly to blame, since the safeguards against self-reactive cells (shaded) are less stringent for B than for T cells. Several **'autoimmune diseases'** are thought to be due to the effects of autoantibodies, mediated via complement, K cells, etc, or indirectly via complexes. Occasionally self-reactivity can be traced to a lack of tolerance to antigens normally sequestered from contact with lymphocytes (column 5) or to non-specific lymphocyte activation (column 6), but usually the cause is unknown; some immunologists regard all autoimmune diseases as secondary to infection or drugs, while others consider autoantibody as a normal part of the disposal of damaged material, and autoimmunity as a failure to regulate this. The old idea that autoantibodies were new 'mutant' antibodies (column 7) is out of fashion, because they are so seldom monoclonal.

Understanding of autoimmunity has been advanced by animal experiments, in particular: (a) the induction of autoantibody in normal animals by cross-reacting ('part-self') antigens, assumed to be due to cooperation between self-reactive B and non-self-reactive T cells (column 4), and (b) spontaneous autoimmune diseases in inbred strains of animals, notably the NZB mouse and the OS chicken, which reveal a multiplicity of genetic influences, at the level of B cells, suppressor T cells, macrophages, target tissues, and hormones (autoimmunity is much commoner and more severe in females).

Viruses, especially those which bud from cells, become associated with MHC antigens (in the mouse, D and K: see Fig 17), and the combination is recognised by cytotoxic T cells. Other viruses, such as influenza, may attach to red cells and induce autoantibody.

Drugs frequently bind to blood cells, either directly (e.g. sedormid to platelets; penicillin to RBC) or as complexes with antibody (e.g. stibophen, PAS, quinidine); antibodies to the drug then destroy the cell. The case of αmethyl dopa is different in that the antibodies are against cell antigens, usually of the Rhesus blood group system, towards which B-cell tolerance is particularly unstable.

Cross-reacting antigens shared between host and microbe may cause autoantibody provided T cells can recognise the non-self and B cells the self (S) determinants. Heteroantigens (e.g. rat thyroglobulin or rat RBC in mice) work in the same way.

Sequestered antigens are assumed not to be 'seen' by lymphocytes until released by organ damage (e.g. eye injury; mumps orchitis). Some intracellular antigens (e.g. after cardiac infarction) may be examples of the same thing.

Adjuvants especially mycobacteria (e.g. Complete Freund's) and endotoxins, can induce autoreactivity by direct lymphocyte stimulation or possibly by inhibiting suppressor cells. In rats, CFA alone can cause arthritis and other diseases with a T-cell element, possibly partly through lymphokine stimulation.

Mutation of antibody combining sites (i.e. 'somatic') was Burnet's original hypothesis of autoimmunity. If valid at all, it is likely to apply only to cases of monoclonal or oligoclonal autoantibody, which, though rare, do occur (e.g. some cold haemolytic anaemias).

Autoantibodies are found in numerous conditions, often being clearly effect rather than cause (e.g. syphilis). But in some diseases they are the first, major, or only detectable abnormality; some of the best-known are listed below:

Haemolytic anaemia and **thrombocytopaenia**, though they can be due to drugs, are more often idiopathic. The correlation between autoantibody levels and cell destruction is not always very close, suggesting another pathological process at work.

Thyroiditis is one of the best candidates for 'primary' autoimmunity. There may be stimulation (thyrotoxicosis) by antibody against the receptor for pituitary TSH, or inhibition (myxoedema) by cell destruction, probably mediated by K cells and autoantibody.

Pernicious anaemia results from a deficiency of gastric Intrinsic Factor, the normal carrier for Vitamin B12. This can be caused both by autoimmune destruction of the parietal cells (atrophic gastritis) and by autoantibodies to Intrinsic Factor itself.

Addison's disease (adrenal hypofunction), **diabetes**, and other endocrine diseases, are often found together in patients or families with thyroid or gastric autoimmunity, suggesting an underlying genetic predisposition.

Myaesthenia gravis, in which neuro-muscular transmission is intermittently defective, is associated with autoantibodies to, and destruction of, the post-synaptic acetyl choline receptors. There are often thymic abnormalities, and thymectomy may be curative, though it is not really clear why.

Rheumatoid arthritis is characterised by, and may be due to, autoantibody against IgG, the joint damage being probably mediated via immune complexes. In this and other autoimmune diseases, the strong association with particular MHC antigens, especially at the D locus, suggests that cell-surface recognition plays a basic initiating role.

SLE In systemic lupus erythematosus the autoantibodies are against DNA and RNA, and the resulting immune complex deposition is widespread throughout the vascular system, giving rise to a 'non-organ-specific' pattern of disease. Like the 'organ specific' diseases (above), non-organ specific diseases tend to occur together. It is not clear why different complexes damage different organs; a localising role for the antigen itself is an obvious possibility.

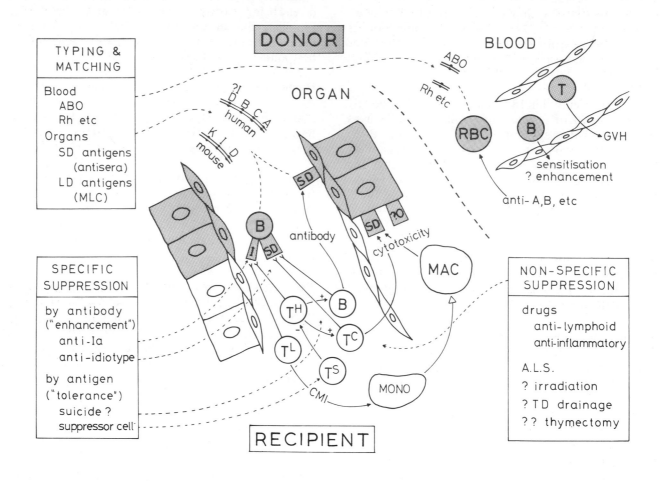

The success of organ grafts between identical ('syngenic'*) twins, and their rejection in all other cases, reflects the remarkable strength of immunological recognition of cell-surface antigens within a species. This is an unfortunate (and in the evolutionary sense unforeseeable) result of the specialisation of T cells for detecting **alterations of MHC antigens**, upon which the response to viruses largely depends (see Figs 17, 21), plus the high degree of **MHC polymorphism** (different antigens in different individuals), which presumably helps a species to maximise its responsive range. Differences in red-cell ('blood-group') antigens also give trouble in blood transfusion (top right) because of antibody; here the rationale for polymorphism is less obvious, but it is much more restricted (e.g. six ABO phenotypes compared to over 10^4 for MHC). The 'minor'

histocompatibility and blood-group antigens appear to be both less polymorphic and antigenically weaker.

Graft rejection can be mediated by T and/or B cells, with their usual non-specific effector adjuncts (complement, K cells, macrophages etc), depending on the target: antibody destroys cells free in the blood, and reacts with vascular endothelium (e.g. of a grafted organ: centre) to initiate Type III inflammation, while T cells attack solid tissue directly or via macrophages. Unless the recipient is already sensitised to donor antigens, these processes do not take effect for a week or more.

Successful organ grafting relies at present on (top left) matching donor and recipient MHC antigens as far as possible (relatives and especially siblings are more likely to share these), and (bottom right) suppressing the residual immune response. The ideal would be (bottom left) to induce specific unresponsiveness to MHC antigens, but this is still experimental (see Immunosuppression, Fig 32).

* Terminology: *syn*genic, *syn*graft: between genetically identical individuals; *allo*- (formerly *homo*-) non-identical, within species; *xeno*- between species; *auto*- same individual.

TYPING AND MATCHING

For blood transfusion, the principle is simple: **A** and/or **B** antigens are detected by agglutination with specific antisera; this is always necessary because normal individuals have antibody against whichever antigen they lack. **Rh** (rhesus) antigens are also typed to avoid sensitising women to those which a prospective child might carry, since Rh incompatibilty can cause serious haemolytic disease in the foetus. Minor antigens only cause trouble in patients sensitised by repeated transfusions. Other possible consequences of blood transfusion are **sensitisation** against MHC antigens carried on B cells, and, in severely immunodeficient patients, **GVH** (graft-versus-host) reactions by transfused T cells against host antigens. The latter is a major complication of bone-marrow grafting.

For organ (e.g. kidney) grafting, MHC antigens must be typed (as well as ABO). Those which elicit antibody responses (**SD**: serologically determined; A, B and C in the human; D and K in the mouse) are detected by agglutination or complement-mediated lysis of B cells or platelets, using antisera from women after childbirth, absorbed to make them monospecific. Those which stimulate lymphocytes (LD: D in the human, I in the mouse — which are probably analogous) are detected by mixed lymphocyte culture (**MLC**) using inducer cells treated to prevent them responding, so that the reaction is 'one-way'.

The success of kidney grafting is related to the degree of match at both SD and LD loci, but not as closely as it should be if these are the only antigens that matter. Minor histocompatibility antigens, perhaps including some restricted to a particular organ (**0** in Figure) may be cumulatively to blame, or there may be another strong locus as yet undetected. With liver grafts, MHC matching has rather less influence on survival, and in some experimental models surprisingly strong tolerance develops. Other organs which survive better than expected include parathyroids and pancreatic Islets.

REJECTION

Taking a kidney graft as typical, rejection can be classified as **immediate**, due to ABO mismatch or MHC presensitisation, **acute** (weeks to months) due to antibody or T-cell responses to MHC antigens, or **chronic** (months to years) usually due to immune complex deposition; it must be remembered that kidney grafting is mainly done to replace organs themselves damaged by immune complex disease. However, many kidneys survive, with the help of immunosuppressive drugs, and some degree of

Rejection continued

tolerance may even develop. Despite the risk of sensitisation, there is evidence that blood transfusion may actually improve graft survival, perhaps by inducing enhancing antibodies. On the other hand, it is claimed that depleting an organ graft of its lymphocytes (e.g. by culture or irradiation) reduces the immune response it induces.

Grafts that are not vascularised (cornea, cartilage) do not normally immunise the recipient and are allowed the 'privilege' of survival. Why the normal foetus is not rejected is still something of a mystery, despite evidence for a number of possible mechanisms, including specific suppressor cells, serum blocking and immunosuppressive factors, and special properties of both placenta (maternal) and trophoblast (foetal).

IMMUNOSUPPRESSION
(see Fig 32 for further details)

Non-specific suppression of lymphocyte division by cytotoxic drugs, together with the anti-inflammatory effects of steroids, are the mainstay of post operative treatment.

ALS Anti-lymphocyte serum, sometimes used in the hope of avoiding damage to dividing non-lymphoid cells (bone marrow; gut).

TD (thoracic duct) drainage and **thymectomy** are occasionally used to deplete T cells.

Irradiation Whole-body X-irradiation is highly immunosuppressive, and local irradiation (e.g. of a kidney) or extracorporeal irradiation of blood to destroy lymphocytes, are sometimes used in acute rejection crises.

Specific suppression is directed at either the antigens inducing a response or the receptors on the cells carrying it out. When brought about by antibody, this is conventionally called **enhancement** and when by antigen, **tolerance**.

Suicide of specific T and B cells can be induced *in vitro* by letting them bind lethal (e.g. radioactive or drug-coupled) antigen.

Suppressor cells or antibodies, by mimicking normal 'network' control, might lead to stable tolerance.

32 Immunosuppression

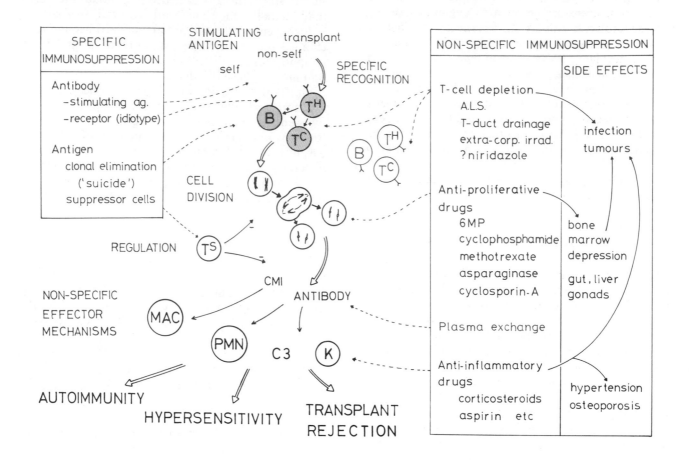

Suppression of immune responses, a regular part of the management of organ transplantation, can also be of value in cases of severe hypersensitivity and auto-immunity. Most of the methods currently available are more or less non-specific, and their use is limited by dangerous side-effects (right).

The problem is to interfere with specific T and/or B cells (top centre, shaded) or their effects, without causing damage to other vital functions. T cells can be **depleted** by anti-lymphocyte antisera (ALS) and by removing or damaging recirculating cells (which are mostly T); however this will remove not only undesirable lymphocytes but others upon whose normal response to infection life may depend (**B, T** unshaded). Lymphocytes almost always divide in the course of responding to antigen (centre), so drugs which inhibit **cell division** are effective immunosuppressants (the same drugs tend to be useful in treating cancer for the same reason); here the danger is that other dividing tissues, such as bone marrow and intestinal epithelium, will also be inhibited. A third point of attack is the **non-specific effector mechanisms** involved in the 'inflammatory' pathways (bottom) which so often cause the actual damage, but here again useful and harmful elements are knocked out indiscriminately.

What is clearly needed is an attack focussed on antigen-specific lymphocytes — that is, an attack via their receptors (top left). This might take the form of masking the antigens they are stimulated by, masking or removing the receptors themselves, or using them to deliver a 'suicidal' dose of antigen to the cell. Whether any of these experimental approaches will be effective enough to replace the present clumsy but well-tried methods of immunosuppression, time will tell.

ALS (anti-lymphocyte serum) is made by immunising horses or rabbits with human lymphocytes and absorbing out unwanted specificities. It depletes especially T cells, probably largely by opsonising them for phagocytosis. It has found a limited use in organ transplantation.

Extracorporeal irradiation of blood, and **thoracic duct drainage** are drastic measures to deplete recirculating T cells, occasionally used in transplant rejection crises.

Niridazole, originally an anthelminthic drug, inhibits T-cell responses, but the mechanism is not known.

6MP (6-mercaptopurine) and its precursor **azathioprine**, block purine metabolism, which is needed for DNA synthesis; despite side-effects on bone marrow polymorph and platelet production, they are standard therapy in organ transplantation and widely used in autoimmune diseases, e.g. rheumatoid arthritis and SLE.

Cyclophosphamide and **chlorambucil** are 'alkylating' agents, which cross-link the DNA strands and prevent them replicating properly. Cyclophosphamide tends to affect B cells more than T, and there is some evidence that it also acts on Ig receptor renewal. It is effective in autoimmune diseases where antibody is a major factor (rheumatoid arthritis, SLE), but the common side-effect of sterility limits its use to older patients.

Methotrexate, Fluorodeoxyuridine, and **Cytosine arabinoside** are other examples of drugs inhibiting DNA synthesis by interfering with various pathways, which have been considered as possible immunosuppressives.

Asparaginase, a bacterial enzyme, starves dividing lymphocytes (and tumour cells) of asparagine, bone marrow etc being spared.

Cyclosporin A is an interesting new immunosuppressive agent obtained from a fungus. It appears to destroy only dividing T and B cells, and has proved remarkably effective in experimental organ transplantation, but unfortunately shows some toxicity towards the kidney.

Plasma exchange, in which blood is removed and the cells separated from the plasma, and returned in dextran or some other plasma substitute, has been successful in acute crises of myaesthenia gravis, Goodpastures's syndrome, and SLE, by reducing (usually only transiently) the level of circulating antibody or complexes.

Corticosteroids (e.g. cortisone, prednisone) are, together with azathioprene, the mainstay of organ transplant immunosuppression, and are also valuable in almost all hypersensitivity and autoimmune diseases. They may act on T cells, but their main effect is probably on polymorph and macrophage activity. Sodium retention ($\rightarrow$ hypertension)) and calcium loss ($\rightarrow$ osteoporosis) are the major undesirable side effects.

Aspirin, indomethacin, and a variety of other antiflammatory drugs are useful in autoimmune diseases with an inflammatory component.

SPECIFIC IMMUNOSUPPRESSION

Regardless of the underlying mechanism, specific suppression mediated by antibody is traditionally known as 'enhancement' and that induced by antigen as 'tolerance'; however, since injection of antigen may often work by inducing antibody, both terms are better replaced, whenever possible, by a description of what is actually happening.

Antibody against **target antigens**, which is especially effective in preventing rejection of tumours, probably works by blocking Ia determinants (see Fig 31). Anti-Rhesus (D) antibodies will prevent sensitisation of Rh-negative mothers in the same way.

Antibody against **receptor idiotypes**, both B and T, might theoretically block recognition of antigen. Whether this block would be self-maintaining enough to be useful in transplantation or autoimmunity is uncertain.

Clonal elimination, or 'classical tolerance' can be induced *in vitro* by coupling cytotoxic drugs or radio-isotopes to antigen, which is then concentrated on the surface of those cells specifically binding it; some success has also been obtained *in vivo* with this 'retiarian therapy' (named after the Roman warriors who caught their victim with a net and then killed him with a spear). It is quite possible that the suppression caused by antiproliferative drugs (e.g. cyclophosphamide, cyclosporin A) in the presence of antigen, contains an element of specific clonal elimination.

Suppressor cells have been found in occasional successful transplant models, and are thought to be lacking in some autoimmune diseases (see Fig 30), but there is no guaranteed method of inducing them to order.

33 Immunodeficiency

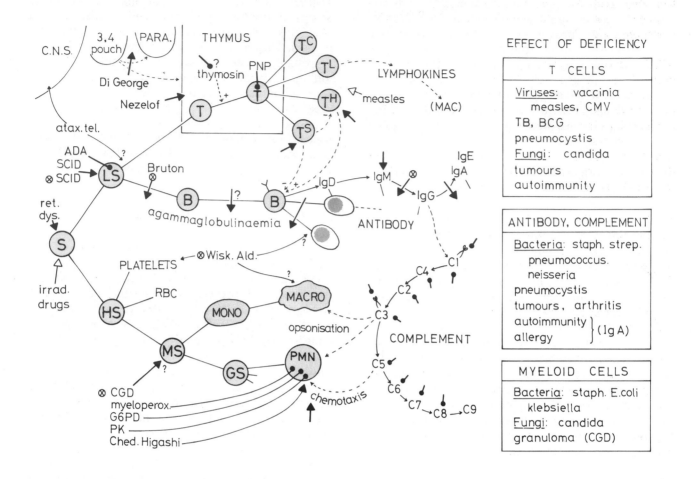

EFFECT OF DEFICIENCY

T CELLS
Viruses: vaccinia measles, CMV
TB, BCG
pneumocystis
Fungi: candida
tumours
autoimmunity

ANTIBODY, COMPLEMENT
Bacteria: staph. strep. pneumococcus. neisseria
pneumocystis
tumours, arthritis
autoimmunity allergy } (IgA)

MYELOID CELLS
Bacteria: staph. E.coli klebsiella
Fungi: candida
granuloma (CGD)

Satisfactory immunity depends on the interaction of such an enormous variety of factors, that inevitably a corresponding variety of different **defects** can reduce its efficiency, all with much the same end-result: increased susceptibility to infection (right). There is a tendency for somewhat different patterns of disease according to whether the defect predominantly affects T cells (top), antibody and/or complement (centre) or myeloid cells (bottom).

Immunodeficiency may be **secondary** to other conditions (e.g. drugs, malnutrition, or infection itself), or due to **primary** genetic defects. It is remarkable how many of the latter are 'X-linked' (i.e. inherited by boys from their mothers; ⊗ in figure), suggesting that the unpaired part of the X chromosome carries several immunologically important genes. In some cases it appears that cell differentiation is interrupted at a particular stage (black arrows), but much more often there is a variable mixture of partial and apparently disconnected defects. In a few diseases the missing gene product can be identified (e.g. individual complement components, polymorph or lymphocyte enzymes (black circles)), and it is to be hoped that this list will grow — not only for the sake of proper classification on a biochemical basis, but because of the possibility of replacement therapy.

The incidence of immunodeficiency depends on the definition of normality. Some form of obvious deficiency is found in more than one person per 1000, but this is clearly an underestimate, judging by the frequency with which 'normal' people succumb periodically to colds, sore throats, boils, etc. In fact the immunological basis of *minor* ill-health is a field whose surface has hardly yet been scratched.

(For details of cellular development and nomenclature, see Figs 4 and 9)

DEFECTS AFFECTING SEVERAL TYPES OF CELL

Ret. dys reticular dysgenesis, a complete failure of stem cells, not compatible with survival for more than a few days after birth.

SCID severe combined immunodeficiency, in which both T and B cells are defective. Some cases are X-linked, and others appear to be due to deficiency of an enzyme, adenosine deaminase (**ADA**), which can be replaced by blood or marrow transfusion.

Atax. tel ataxia telangectasia, a combination of defects in brain, skin, T cells and immunoglobulin (especially IgA).

Wisk. Ald Wiskott-Aldrich syndrome, another strange combination with eczema, platelet deficiency, and absent antibody response to polysaccharides (perhaps a B-cell subpopulation defect?).

DEFECTS PREDOMINANTLY AFFECTING T CELLS

Di George syndrome; absence of thymus and parathyroids, with maldevelopment of other 3rd and 4th pharyngeal pouch derivatives. Serious but very rare, it may respond to thymus grafting.

Nezelof syndrome; somewhat similar to Di George but with normal parathyroids.

PNP purine nucleoside phosphorylase, a purine salvage enzyme found in T cells. Deficiency causes nucleosides, particularly deoxyguanosine, to accumulate and damage the T cell. Interestingly, at low concentrations of deoxyguanosine, suppressor T cells are more sensitive than other types.

Measles infection is particularly liable to suppress T-cell function. In all cases of T-cell deficiency, cell-mediated responses are of course reduced, but there are often secondary effects on antibody as well.

DEFECTS PREDOMINANTLY AFFECTING B CELLS

Agammaglobulinaemia or hypogammaglobulinaemia may reflect the absence of B cells (Bruton type), their failure to differentiate into plasma cells (variable types), or selective inability to make one class of immunoglobulin — most commonly IgA, but sometimes IgG or IgM. Some cases may be due to abnormalities of T helper or suppressor cells.

Defects predominantly affecting B cells continued

Autoimmunity, allergies, and polyarthritis, are remarkably common in patients with antibody deficiencies, while both T and B-cell defects appear to increase the risk of tumours (see Fig 25).

DEFECTS OF COMPLEMENT

Virtually all the complement components may be genetically deficient; sometimes there is complete absence, sometimes a greatly reduced level, suggesting a regulatory rather than a structural gene defect. In addition, deficiency of inactivators may cause trouble, e.g. C1 inhibitor (hereditary angio-oedema); C3b inhibitor (KAF; very low C3 levels).

DEFECTS AFFECTING MYELOID CELLS

CGD chronic granulomatous disease, an X-linked defect of peroxide production, leading to chronic infection with bacteria that do not themselves produce peroxide (catalase positive). There may be other abnormalities, and monocytes are also affected, suggesting a defect in a common precursor cell.

Myeloperoxidase, G6PD (glucose-6-phosphate dehydrogenase), **PK** (pyruvate kinase) and no doubt other polymorph enzymes may be genetically deficient, causing recurrent infection with bacteria and sometimes fungi.

Ched. Higashi In the Chediak-Higashi syndrome, the polymorphs contain large granules but do not form proper phagolysosomes. In other cases the response to chemotaxis is impaired ('lazy leucocyte').

SECONDARY IMMUNODEFICIENCY

Age Immunity tends to be weaker in infancy and old age — the former being partly compensated by passively transferred maternal antibody.

Malnutrition is associated with defects in antibody and, in severe cases, T cells; this may explain the more serious course of diseases (e.g. measles) in tropical countries. Both calorie and protein intake are important, as well as minerals such as iron and zinc.

Tumours are often associated with immunodeficiency, notably Hodgkin's disease, myeloma, and leukaemias; it is sometimes hard to be sure which is cause and which effect. The same is true for the immunodeficiency of infections.

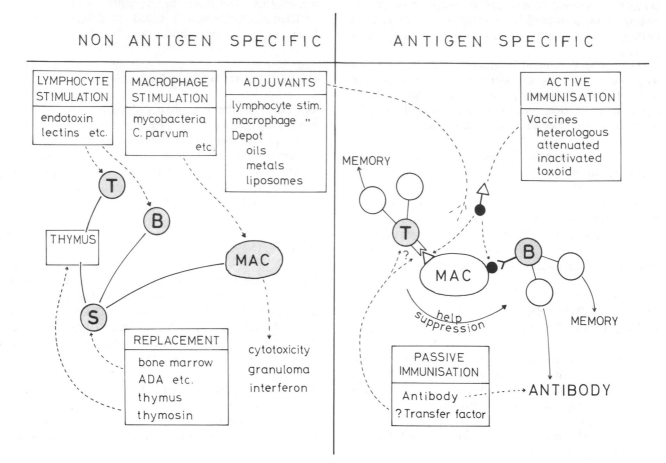

NON ANTIGEN SPECIFIC | ANTIGEN SPECIFIC

LYMPHOCYTE STIMULATION
endotoxin
lectins etc.

MACROPHAGE STIMULATION
mycobacteria
C. parvum
etc.

ADJUVANTS
lymphocyte stim.
macrophage "
Depot
  oils
  metals
  liposomes

ACTIVE IMMUNISATION
Vaccines
  heterologous
  attenuated
  inactivated
  toxoid

THYMUS

MEMORY

T   B   MAC   S

REPLACEMENT
bone marrow
ADA etc.
thymus
thymosin

cytotoxicity
granuloma
interferon

T   MAC   B

help
suppression

MEMORY

PASSIVE IMMUNISATION
Antibody
?Transfer factor

ANTIBODY

In most animals the combination of natural resistance and stimulation of adaptive responses by antigen is adequate to cope with common infections, otherwise the species would not survive. However the immune system does have its shortcomings, some of which can be overcome by artificial means.

Natural immune mechanisms generally act, against a given challenge, either briskly or not at all. But there are times when they appear to be on the brink of success (e.g. against some tumours and parasites), and when it may be possible to tip the balance by **non-specific immunostimulation** (top left).

Adaptive immune responses, on the other hand, suffer from their initial slowness, so that high levels of antibody may arrive too late to prevent death or disability (e.g. tetanus, polio), though surviving patients are resistant to reinfection. Here **specific**

immunisation is usually the answer; this may be **active** (top right), in which antigen is used to safely generate immunological memory, aided in some cases by the boosting power of special non-specific stimulants or **adjuvants**, or **passive**, in which preformed antibody is injected, with more rapid but short-lived effect.

Finally, when some component of the immune system is deficient (see Fig 33), efforts can be made to correct this by **replacement** of hormones, enzymes, cells, or organs (bottom left). As knowledge grows, replacement of the defective gene will probably take the place of these temporising measures. Meanwhile, new immunostimulants are constantly being reported, and the possibility that some apparently irrational remedy may benefit the immune system in ways at present unmeasurable, should never be hastily dismissed.

REPLACEMENT THERAPY

S. Stem cells; in some cases of severe combined immunodeficiency, bone marrow grafting has restored function; where adenosine deaminase (**ADA**) is deficient, this enzyme may also be restored by blood transfusion.

Thymus grafting has been effective in restoring T-cell function in the Di George syndrome. Thymic extracts (e.g. 'thymosin') have been tried in a number of T-cell deficient states.

LYMPHOCYTE STIMULATION

Numerous substances non-specifically stimulate lymphocytes to divide ('mitogens') and exert their usual function ('polyclonal activation'); often these act predominantly on one cell type, e.g. bacterial endotoxins (LPS) and polyanions (dextran sulphate) affect B cells, while Levamisole, Lentinan, double-stranded RNA, and the lectin Concanavalin A affect mainly T cells. Often the same substance can stimulate or suppress an immune response, depending on the precise timing of administration.

MACROPHAGE STIMULATION

Mycobacteria (e.g. BCG) **Corynebacteria**, and some of the lymphocyte stimulators listed above, can 'activate' macrophages, the most useful result being to increase their antitumour effect, probably by stimulating both local cytotoxicity and the secretion of factors. Activated macrophages are also more effective against intracellular bacteria and protozoa, and (via interferon secretion) viruses.

ADJUVANTS

Adjuvants are materials which increase the response to a simultaneously administered antigen. It is not known exactly how any adjuvant works, but stimulation of T cells, B cells, and macrophages are a common feature (most of the above-mentioned agents have adjuvant properties) and there is an additional group of substances which bind or retain antigen, improving and prolonging its antigenicity; these include oil emulsions, metal salts (e.g. $Al(OH)_3$), and more recently synthetic lipid vesicles ('liposomes'). The most powerful adjuvants (e.g. Freund's Complete) combine several of these properties. Unfortunately the latter is too tissue-destructive for human use, and considerable efforts are being made to find safer adjuvants. Various defined fractions of mycobacterial cell walls and their synthetic analogues seem to offer the best hope at present, but the problem is far from solved.

The term 'vaccine', introduced by Pasteur to commemorate Jenner's classic work with cowpox (vaccinia), is loosely applied to all agents used to induce specific immunity and mitigate the effects of subsequent infection. Vaccines are given as early as practical, taking into account the fact that the immune system is not fully developed in the first months of life, and that antibody passively acquired from the mother via the placenta and/or milk will specifically prevent the baby making his own response. In general this means a first injection at about 6 months, with subsequent boosts, but precise schedules may depend on the local prevalence of particular diseases, and can be found in specialised textbooks.

Heterologous vaccines work by producing a milder but cross-protecting disease, the only common example being vaccinia, which has effectively allowed the elimination of smallpox.

Attenuated viruses (measles, yellow fever, polio (Sabin), rubella) or bacteria (BCG) produce subclinical disease and usually excellent protection. Care is needed, however, in immunodeficient patients.

Inactivated vaccines are used where attenuation is not feasible; they include formalin-killed viruses such as rabies and influenza, and bacteria such as cholera and pertussis (whooping cough). Killed vaccines are safer but usually less effective than live ones, though some of them may have a useful adjuvant effect on other vaccines given with them (e.g. pertussis in the 'triple vaccine' with diptheria and tetanus).

Toxoids are bacterial toxins (e.g. diptheria, tetanus) inactivated with formalin but still antigenic. Other subcellular fractions (e.g. the capsular polysaccharides of meningococci) can also induce protective antibody.

PASSIVE IMMUNISATION

Antibody In patients already exposed to disease, passively transferred antiserum may be life-saving; examples are tetanus, hepatitis B, snakebite. Originally antisera were raised in horses, but the danger of serum sickness (see Fig 28) makes convalescent human serum preferable. In patients with antibody deficiency, normal human gammaglobulin provides good protection against common infections.

Transfer factor an extract of normal leucocytes, was originally thought to transfer specific immuno-competence to T cells, but there are now doubts about the specificity. Nevertheless in some infections, despite the lack of rationale (as so often in immunology) it does seem to work.

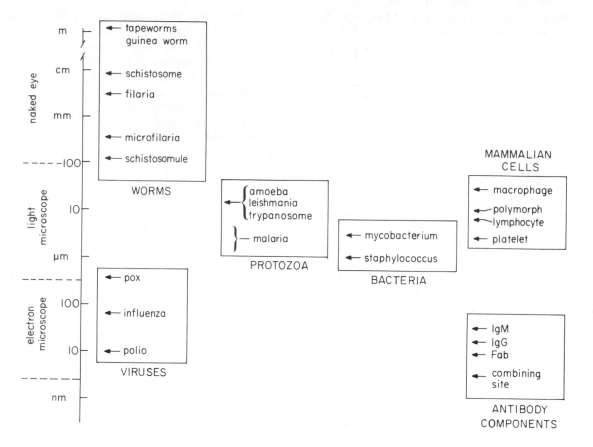

Comparative Molecular Weights

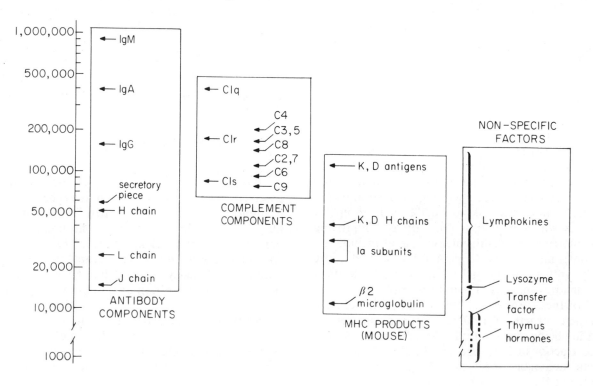

1798	Jenner: vaccination against smallpox: the beginning of immunology.		1944-	Medawar: skin graft rejection as an immune response.
1881-5	Pasteur: attenuated vaccines (cholera, anthrax, rabies).		1945	Coombs: anti-globulin test for red-cell autoantibody.
1882	Metchnikoff: phagocytosis (in starfish).		1947	Owen: tolerance in cattle twins.
1888	Roux; Yersin: diphtheria antitoxin (antibody).		1952	Bruton: agammaglobulinaemia.

1798 Jenner: vaccination against smallpox: the beginning of immunology.
1881-5 Pasteur: attenuated vaccines (cholera, anthrax, rabies).
1882 Metchnikoff: phagocytosis (in starfish).
1888 Roux; Yersin: diphtheria antitoxin (antibody).
1890 Von Behring: passive protection (tetanus) by antibody.
1891 Koch: delayed hypersensitivity (tuberculosis).
1893 Buchner: heat labile serum factor (complement).
1896 Widal: diagnosis by antibody (typhoid).
1897 Ehrlich: 'side chain' (receptor) theory.
1900 Landsteiner: ABO groups in blood transfusion.
1902 Portier & Richet: hypersensitivity.
1903 Arthus: local anaphylaxis.
1906 Von Pirquet: allergy.
1910 Dale: histamine.
1917- Landsteiner: haptens, carriers, and antibody specificity.
1922 Fleming: lysozyme.
1938 Tiselius & Kabat: antibodies as gamma-globulins.
1943 Chase: transfer of delayed hypersensitivity by cells.

1944- Medawar: skin graft rejection as an immune response.
1945 Coombs: anti-globulin test for red-cell autoantibody.
1947 Owen: tolerance in cattle twins.
1952 Bruton: agammaglobulinaemia.
1953 Billingham, Brent & Medawar: neonatal induction of tolerance.
1956 Glick: bursa dependence of antibody response.
1956 Roitt & Doniach: autoantibodies in thyroid disease.
1957 Isaacs: interferon.
1959 Porter; Edelman: enzyme cleavage of antibody molecule.
1959 Gowans: lymphocyte recirculation.
1959 Burnet: clonal selection theory.
1960 Nowell: lymphocyte transformation (PHA).
1961-2 Miller; Good: thymus dependence of immune responses.
1966-7 Claman; Davies; Mitchison: T-B cell cooperation.
1971 Gershon: suppression by T cells.
1974 Jerne: network theory of immune regulation.
1975 Zinkernagel & Doherty; Bevan: dual recognition by T cells.
1975 Köhler & Milstein; monoclonal antibodies from hybridomas.

Some unsolved problems

Antibody: how many germ line genes and how much somatic diversification?

Cancer: will immunology help?

HLA and disease: how and why are they associated?

Human organ grafting: what are the critical antigens and will specific tolerance be possible?

Networks: how important are they in regulating immune responses and can they be exploited to control them?

T cells: what is their receptor and how does it acquire specificity?

Thymus hormones: are they real and will they be useful?

Transfer factor: what is it and how does it work?

Vaccination: will the parasite diseases succumb?

Index

Page numbers in bold type indicate the figures on which principal references appear